Manual of
Hysteroscopy

61st AICOG 2018 Odisha

61st AICOG BHUBANESWAR 2018

Manual of
Hysteroscopy

Editors

SN Tripathy

KC Mahapatra

SK Giri

Sunita Tandulwadkar

Sujata Swain

61st AICOG Odisha 2018

61st AICOG BHUBANESWAR 2018

JAYPEE *The Health Sciences Publisher*

New Delhi | London | Panama

Jaypee Brothers Medical Publishers (P) Ltd

Headquarters
Jaypee Brothers Medical Publishers (P) Ltd
4838/24, Ansari Road, Daryaganj
New Delhi 110 002, India
Phone: +91-11-43574357
Fax: +91-11-43574314
Email: jaypee@jaypeebrothers.com

Overseas Offices

J.P. Medical Ltd
83 Victoria Street, London
SW1H 0HW (UK)
Phone: +44-20 317 08910
Fax: +44 (0)20 3008 6180
Email: info@jpmedpub.com

Jaypee-Highlights Medical Publishers Inc
City of Knowledge, Bld. 235, 2nd floor, Clayton
Panama City, Panama
Phone: +1 507-301-0496
Fax: +1 507-301-0499
Email: cservice@jphmedical.com

Jaypee Brothers Medical Publishers (P) Ltd
17/1-B Babar Road, Block-B, Shyamoli
Mohammadpur, Dhaka-1207
Bangladesh
Mobile: +08801912003485
Email: jaypeedhaka@gmail.com

Jaypee Brothers Medical Publishers (P) Ltd
Bhotahity, Kathmandu, Nepal
Phone: +977-9741283608
Email: Kathmandu@jaypeebrothers.com

Website: www.jaypeebrothers.com
Website: www.jaypeedigital.com

Inquiries for bulk sales may be solicited at: jaypee@jaypeebrothers.com

Manual of Hysteroscopy

First Edition: **2018**

ISBN 978-93-5270-369-2

Printed at: Samrat Offset Pvt. Ltd.

Contributors

Abhishek Chandavarkar
Mumbai, Maharashtra, India

Bhardwaj F

HP Patnaik
Cuttack, Odisha, India

Madhura Chandavarkar

Malvika Sabharwal
Delhi, India

Mittal M

Nahata VS
Mahatma Gandhi Medical College
Jaipur, Rajasthan, India

Nibedita Pani
Department of Anesthesiology
SCB Medical College
Cuttack, Odisha, India

Parul Kotdawala
Kotdawala Women's Clinic
Ellis Bridge
Ahmedabad, Gujarat, India

PC Mahapatra
Professor
SCB Medical College
Cuttack, Odisha, India

Polly Chatterjee
Kolkata, India

Priyanka Suhag

Rabi Narayan Satpathy
Assistant Professor
SCB Medical College
Cuttack, Odisha, India

Rohan Krishnakumar
JK Women Hospital
Mumbai, Maharashtra, India

S Krishnakumar

Srimanta Haldar

Sujata Kar
KCHPL
Bhubaneswar, Odisha, India

Sujata Swain
Associate Professor
SCB Medical College
Cuttack, Odisha, India

Message

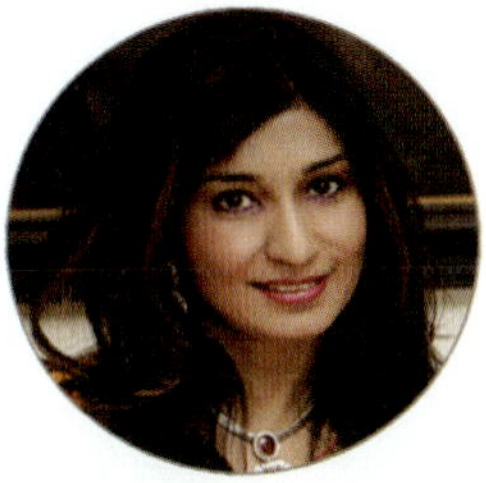

Rishma Dhillon Pai
MD DNB FCPS DGO FICOG
President, FOGSI—2017
Consultant Gynecologist
Jaslok Hospital, Lilavati Hospital and Hinduja Healthcare (Khar),
Bloom IVF Centre,
The Every Woman Clinic,
Mumbai, Maharashtra, India

"Wisdom.... comes not from age, but from education and learning."
Anton Chekhov

Life is a continuous process of learning. Especially in the field of medicine, which is constantly changing, it is very important to keep oneself abreast with the latest developments. It is heartening to note that academic workshop manuals are being released at the AICOG, Bhubaneswar, Odisha, India, for the benefit of the participating delegates and present varied updates in the field. Many different Manuals are being released on important subjects such as *3D Laparoscopy and Operative Oncology, Genetics, Fetal Medicine and Color Doppler, Postpartum Hemorrhage and High-Risk Pregnancy, Hysteroscopy,* etc.

I thank all the authors, for their immense contributions in building up the content for the manuals for Federation of Obstetric and Gynaecological Societies of India (FOGSI) by sharing their rich experiences in the field. These will be a big help to young gynecologists, who are still acquiring skills in various aspects of obstetrics and gynecology and a quick update for the seniors.

I extend congratulations to the organizing team of the AICOG 2018 and the editors of these manuals and wish you all success for this mega event.

"You cannot open a book without learning something."
—Confucius

Message

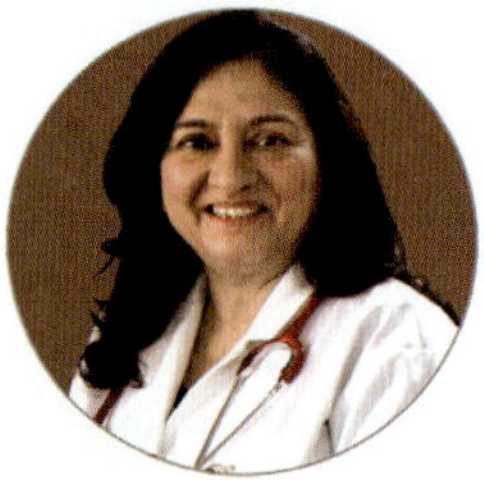

Jaideep Malhotra
MD FICMCH FICS FMAS FRCOG FICOG FRCPI FIAJAGO
Consultant ART (IVF)
President Elect, FOGSI—2018
Director, Rainbow IVF
Agra, Uttar Pradesh, India

"Education is greatest gift of life, it should never stop."

The subject of obstetrics and gynecology needs extreme proficiency as it deals with the medical specialties that focus on two different aspects. First one includes the care of pregnant women, the unborn baby, labor and delivery, as well as the immediate period following childbirth. Second aspect includes dealing with any ailment concerning the female reproductive organs. Hence, the manuals will help all those who are looking forward to gain excellence in the field of woman health. The manuals have tried to address all the issues a doctor needs.

With increasing expertise in all fields, the surgeon therefore while exercising a choice needs to follow the Hippocratic dictum—*"First, do no harm."*

We are thankful to all those who have incorporated their contribution by providing chapters from their research and collected scientific material and have shared their fruitful experiences for the delegates of the workshop.

As a part of my agenda for 2018, I as FOGSI President 2018, plan to work actively on QED (Quality, Ethics and Dignity) among our profession and also work towards HER (Health, Empowerment and Respect) towards our patients.

"Knowledge is of no value unless you put it into practices."

Message

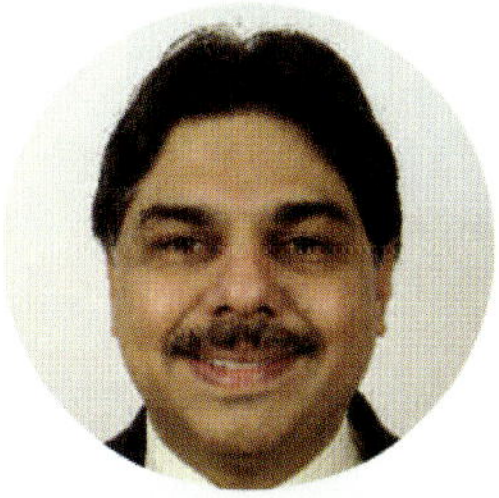

Hrishikesh Pai
Secretary General, FOGSI

It is my proud privilege to invite and welcome all delegates to the 61st All India Congress of Obstetrics and Gynaecology (AICOG) from 17th–21st January, 2018 at the Temple City of India, Bhubaneswar, Odisha, India.

It is propitious to note that the academic workshop manuals are being released which will reap beneficial reward to all the participating delegates.

I thank all the authors, for their immense contributions in building up the content for the manuals for Federation of Obstetric and Gynaecological Societies of India (FOGSI) by sharing their rich experiences in the field. These will be a big help to young gynecologists, who are still acquiring skills in various aspects of obstetrics and gynecology and a quick update for the seniors.

I forward my heartiest congratulations to all the contributors, the editors and the delegates of the workshop.

Message

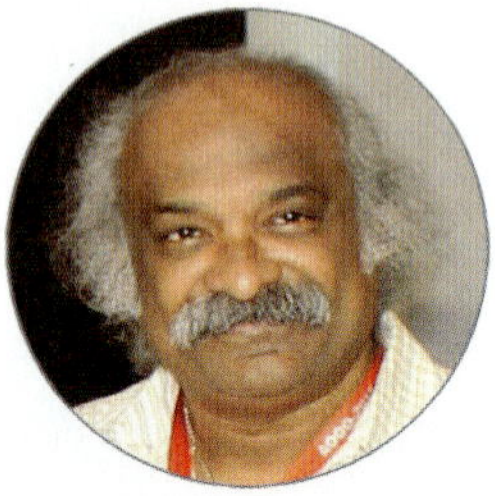

PC Mahapatra
Professor
Department of Obstetrics and Gynecology
SCB Medical College
Cuttack, Odisha, India
President, FOGSI—2011
Organising Chairperson

It is my proud privilege to invite and welcome all delegates to the 61st All India Congress of Obstetrics and Gynaecology (AICOG) from 17th–21st January, 2018 at the Temple City of India, Bhubaneswar, Odisha, India.

The five days of academic extravaganza will certainly enrich the scientific knowledge of all participating delegates and faculty. The precongress workshop on various aspects of this specialty will be held on 17th January 2018.

A quote by Edwin Louis Cole says that "*Winners are not those who never fail but those who never quit*" is apt for all the clinicians who are determined enough to see and overcome all the difficulties that are faced in the field of obstetrics and gynecology.

Today, with the advancement in the field of obstetrics and gynecology, everyone requires an in-depth knowledge of the complex subjects associated with the field so as to gain excellence in it.

This manual will prove to be a boon to all those who are associated with the field and wants to gain more knowledge in the subject matter.

Message

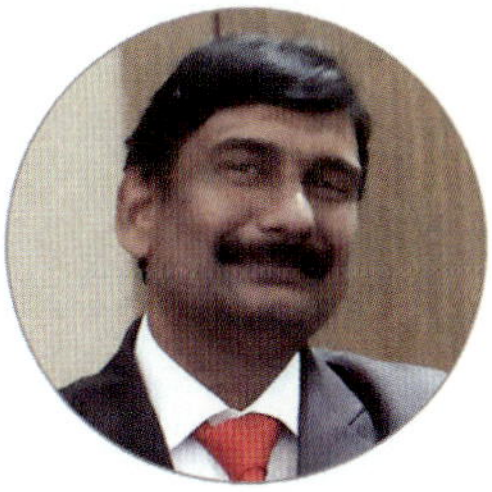

HP Pattanaik
Head
Department of Obstetrics and Gynecology
City Hospital
Cuttack, Odisha, India
Vice President, FOGSI—2009
Organising Secretary

Greetings from 61st AICOG 2018!
It is a matter of great pleasure to invite you all to 61st AICOG, from 17th–21st January, 2018 at the Temple City of India, Bhubaneswar, Odisha, India. The 11th Precongress workshops will be held on 17th January, 2018 in three medical colleges of Bhubaneswar.

It is propitious to note that the academic workshop manuals are being released which will reap beneficial reward to all the participating delegates.

It will also prove to be beneficial to the members of Federation of Obstetric and Gynaecological Societies of India (FOGSI), those who were unable to register themselves for the academic workshops.

I forward my heartiest congratulations to all the contributors, the editors and the delegates of the workshop.

Preface

'The womb is the field of generation; and if this field be corrupted it is in vain to expect any fruit though it be ever so well sown.'

Aristotle

What else is a better method to evaluate the uterus than a hysteroscopc.

Technical and technological advances are continuously revolutionizing our everyday life, at times forcing us to race ahead just to keep up with the times.

Hysteroscopy, although known since 1869 and used since 1925, has gained general acceptance by gynecologists relatively slowly. It was not until 1970 when 32% Dextran was used to distend the uterine cavity, that gynecologists slowly began to utilize hysteroscopy, not only for diagnosis, but also for operative procedures. Many other techniques have subsequently been developed since 1981, when Goldrath and colleagues published data on the use of hysteroscopy to ablate the endometrium with a laser. This opened the gates for the everyday gynecologist to offer alternatives to hysterectomy in the treatment of severe menometrorrhagia. The hysteroscope also permits the outpatient treatment of many other pathologies including submucosal leiomyomas, endometrial polyps, uterine synechia and uterine septa. Recently, hysteroscopic sterilization techniques have been developed and widely accepted as office based procedures.

This book has chapters that address all of the present hysteroscopic therapies and will provide an in depth discussion of the current knowledge of hysteroscopy and global ablation techniques. The reader will note that many topics may appear to be repetitious as the individual chapter authors were allowed to express their views of procedures. There are also some differences in opinion as to techniques. We believe that allowing the freedom to disagree, even in the same book, is in itself, an educational benefit and will expose the reader to a more balanced view of current knowledge. We, the editors, also may not be in complete agreement with some of the views expressed by the chapter authors; however our role is to educate not censor.

'Knoweldge is a flower which never wither.'

Editors

Contents

1. **Operation Theater Setup and Instruments Used in Hysteroscopy** 1
HP Patnaik

2. **Ideal Anesthesia for Hysteroscopy** 13
Nibedita Pani, Srimanta Haldar

3. **Basic Principles in Operative Hysteroscopy** 18
S Krishnakumar, Rohan Krishnakumar

4. **Microhysteroscopy, Contact Hysteroscopy and Office Hysteroscopy** 29
Sujata Swain

5. **Hysteroscopic Evaluation of Infertile Couple** 37
PC Mahapatra

6. **Hysteroscopy in Abnormal Uterine Bleeding** 47
Nahata VS, Bhardwaj F, Mittal M

7. **Hysteroscopic Removal of Intrauterine Contraceptive Devices and Foreign Bodies** 54
Abhishek Chandavarkar, Priyanka Suhag, Madhura Chandavarkar

8. **Role of Hysteroscopy in Müllerian Anomaly** 57
Rabi Narayan Satpathy

9. **Hysteroscopic Myomectomy** 64
Malvika Sabharwal

10. **Transcervical Resection of Uterine Septum** 71
Parul Kotdawala

11. **Complications of Hysteroscopic Surgery** 78
Sujata Kar

12. **Hysteroscopic Contraception** 86
Polly Chatterjee

Chapter 1

Operation Theater Setup and Instruments Used in Hysteroscopy

HP Patnaik

INTRODUCTION

Hysteroscopy is a procedure that involves direct visualization of cervical canal and uterine cavity. Office hysteroscopy allows minor pathologies to be treated in an outpatient setting. Surgical hysteroscopic procedures, or in other words, major hysteroscopic surgery, is performed in the operating room.

Instruments used are (Fig. 1):

- Distending media
- Light source
- Camera
- Telescope
- Diagnostic and operative sheaths
- Accessory instruments.

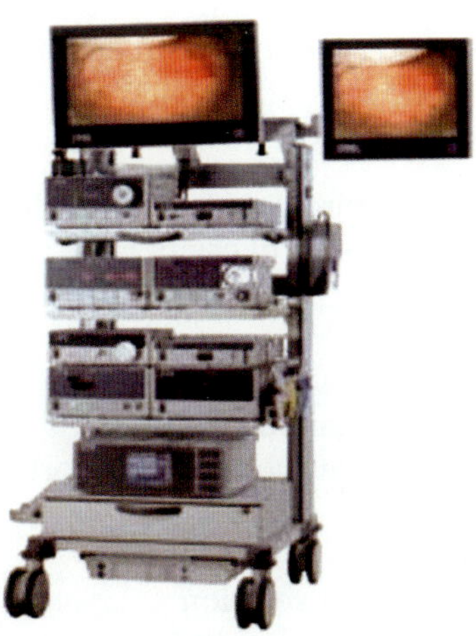

Fig. 1: Fully equipped mobile cart for both diagnostic and surgical hysteroscopy as well as laparoscopy.

MEDIA FOR DISTENDING THE UTERINE CAVITY

All hysteroscopic procedures require adequate distension of the uterine cavity.

Due to office hysteroscopy and the bipolar resectoscope, it is possible to use physiological saline solution as the unique method of distension. Current is strictly limited to the resectoscope's two poles without flowing through the patient's body for high-frequency bipolar intrauterine electrosurgery, hence it is possible to use physiological saline as distension media.[1]

Types

- Gaseous—carbon dioxide (CO_2)
- Liquid
  - High viscosity—Hyskon
  - Low viscosity
- Ionic: NS, RL, 5% D, 10% D, 4% and 6% dextran solution
- Nonionic: 1.5% glycine, 35 sorbitol, 5% mannitol
- Combination of 2.8% sorbitol and 0.5% mannitol.

CO_2 as Distending Media

- Used in office hysteroscopy
- Rate of flow: 30–40 mL/min (should be less than 100 mL/min)
- Intrauterine pressure 60–70 mm Hg.

Advantages

- Provides clean media
- Allows entry evaluation of endocervical canal.

Disadvantages

- Does not flush cavity of debris
- Flattens endometrium
- Emboli can form causing gas embolism and death.[2]

Low Viscosity Distending Media

- Delivered fluid must be circulated out and clear fluid added in order to maintain view and distension of cavity
- Delivery Systems used are:
  - Gravity fall system
  - Pressure cuff
  - Electronic suction irrigation pump.
- Proper monitoring of infused volume is important and infusion is stopped when positive.
- Infusion difference is
  - 500 cc for hypo-osmolar solution
  - 1000 cc for iso-osmolar solution.[2]

Normal Saline

- 0.9% NS is commonly used.

Advantages: Easily available, low operative cost and physiological disposal by peritoneal absorption.

Disadvantages: Efficient conductor of electrons so electrosurgery with monopolar devices is not possible. Not suitable for office hysteroscopy. Fluid overload and pulmonary edema risk.[2]

Glycine (1.5%) and Sorbitol (3%)

Advantages
Inexpensive, easily available, media of choice for monopolar cautery.

Disadvantages
- Hypoosmolar solution causing dilutional hyponatremia and hypervolemia.
- Interferes with oxygenation and coagulation.[3]

Mannitol (5%) and Glycine (2.2%)
- Isosmolar
- Can be used with electrosurgical instruments
- Decreased risk of fluid overload and hyponatremia.

High Viscosity Media––Hyskon
- It is a 32% high molecular weight dextran solution
- Colorless viscid medium
- Volume required: Diagnostic—100 mL, operative—200-500 mL, upper safe limit—500 mL
- One mL of Hyskon withdraws 20 mL of water in circulation.

Advantages
- Being highly viscous small quantities required for examination
- Provides excellent visualization due to high refractive index.

Disadvantages
- Expensive mechanical pump necessary to deliver these fluids
- Pulmonary edema, coagulopathies, electrolyte imbalance, anaphylactic reaction.[3]

LIGHT SOURCE

Quality depends upon:
- Wattage
- Remote light generator
- Structural integrity of light cable.

Wattage

- 175 W for routine procedures
- 300 W for special interventions.

Light Generator

- Tungsten orange yellow light
- Metal halide bluish coloration
  - Xenon white light
  - LED source.[4]

IMAGING SYSTEMS

The use of an endocamera is essential in modern hysteroscopy. Different types of video cameras are available; their quality depends on the following technical parameters: resolution (given by number of lines or pixels), and sensitivity (Lux), as well as the quality of the reproduction or video images. A high signal-to-noise ratio indicates that variations in image quality under extreme situations, e.g. hemorrhages or other reasons for loss of light intensity are reduced to a minimum. Modern high definition (HD) cameras offer a very high resolution and almost natural color reproduction.

TELESCOPE

It has three parts:
- Eyepiece
- Barrel
- Objective lens.

Available in various diameters:
- 4 mm (standard)--gives high quality, sharpest image
- 3 mm—inferior to 4 mm, but gives satisfactory image quality.

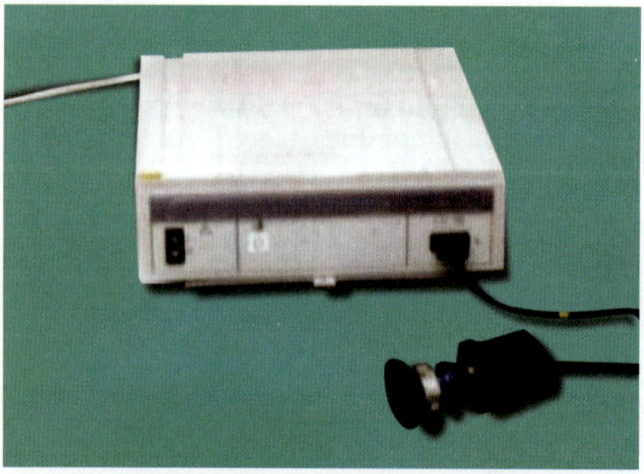

Fig. 2: Telescope.

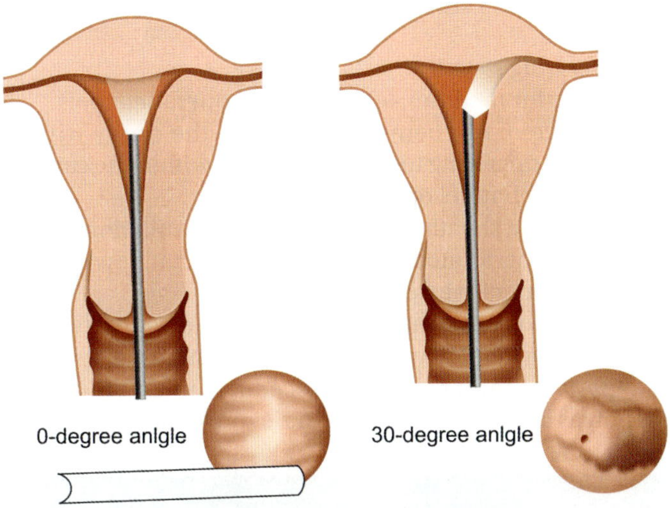

Fig. 3: Hysteroscopic views.

Types

- Straight on, i.e. 0°--distant panoramic view
- Forward-oblique, i.e. 30°--advantage is that by rotating it, all walls and cornual ends can be visualized[3] (Fig. 3).

DIAGNOSTIC SHEATHS

- Usually 4–5 mm
- Required to deliver the distending media into the uterine cavity. Telescope fits into the sheath and there is 1 mm gap left between the sheath and scope through which distending media is transmitted and is controlled by external stopcock. The endoscopes used in this field of application are available in different outer diameters. Miniature endoscopes should be used in diagnostic hysteroscopy in order to render the procedure minimally invasive. Microhysteroscopy is usually performed with a 2 mm telescope, which involves considerable limitations due to fragility of scope. It should be reserved for special cases of cervical stenosis. The hysteroscope with a diameter of 2.9 mm is most widely used in office setting, including purely diagnostic hysteroscopy, using physiological saline as distension media.[1,5]

OPERATIVE HYSTEROSCOPES

It has channels for:

- 3–4 mm telescope
- Instillation of medium
- Operating instruments.

Types

- *Standard operating sheath:*
  - Single cavity for medium, telescope and operating tools.
  - Disadvantage of not being able to flush the cavity with distending medium and operating tool manipulation within the cavity is difficult.
- Isolated multiple channel operating sheath:
  - Double flushing sheath that allows media instillation by inner sheath and return by perforated outer sheath, constant flow of medium leads to very clear operative field.

Operative hysteroscopes have been definitively superseded by office hysteroscopy systems that allow for diagnostic hysteroscopy while providing the option to perform minor surgical procedures in an office setting (small endometrial polyps or pedunculated uterine leiomyomas). For this purpose, the

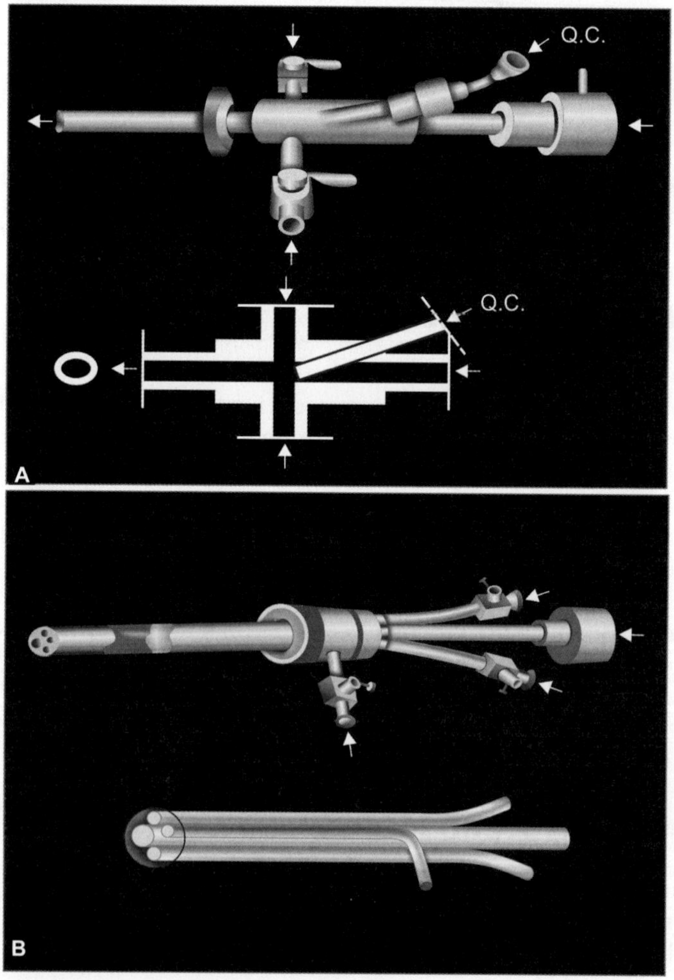

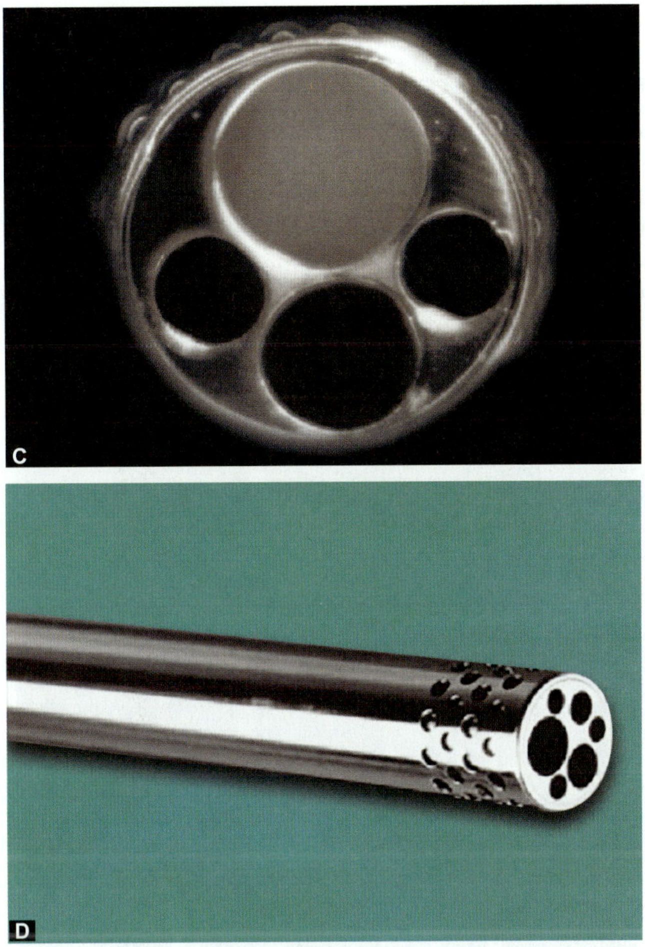

Figs. 4A to D

inner diameter of the sheath used in conjunction with an office hysteroscope must be large enough to permit the passage of operating instruments. Indeed, even if the same telescope is used as in diagnostic hysteroscopy (2.9 mm diameter), the sheath must have an outer diameter ranging between 3.2 mm and 5.3 mm to permit the passage of surgical instruments and to provide adequate uterine distension by use of liquid media. In this field of application, most operating instruments have a semi-rigid design and a diameter of 1.67 mm (5 Fr): scissors, biopsy forceps, and various types of probes, electrodes for unipolar and bipolar coagulation, and Essure microinsert for hysteroscopic sterilization by tubal occlusion in a clinical setting.[1,6]

RESECTOSCOPES

Electrosurgical Endoscope (Fig. 5)

- Consists of:
  - Inner sheath has a common channel for telescope, distending media and electrode.
  - Outer sheath--for the return of distending media.
- Lens is angled towards the electrode for clear view.
  - Electrode can be ball, barrel, knife, or cutting loop type.

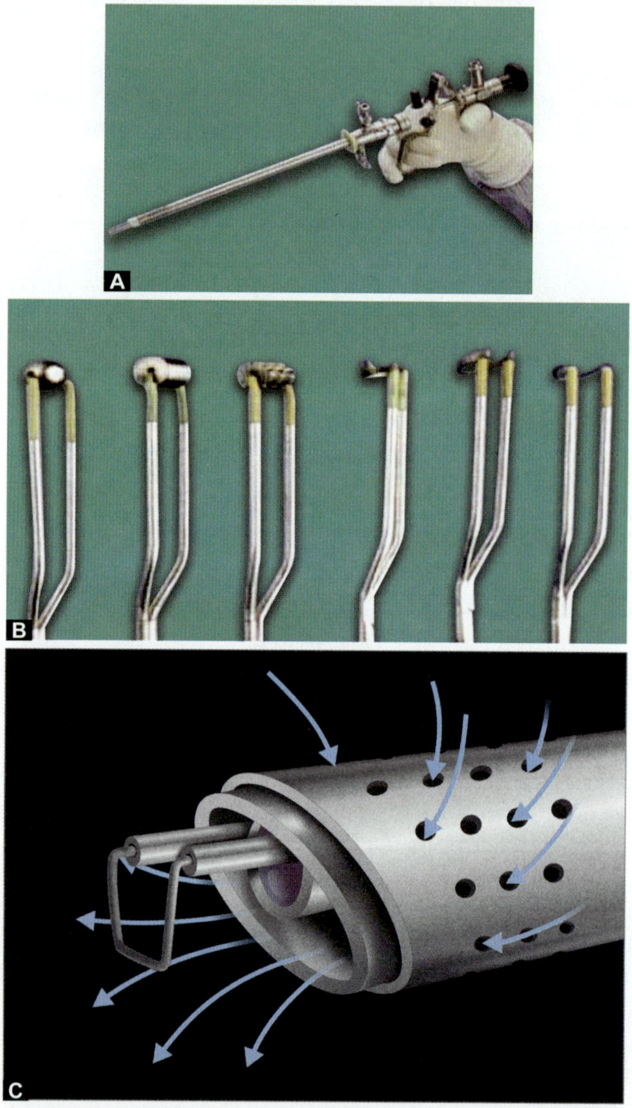

Figs. 5A to C: (A) Resectoscope, (B) Accessories with resectoscope, (C) Distension medium flow through resectoscope.

Resectoscope is specially designed for the resection and removal of abnormal intrauterine tissue as well as endometrial ablation and septal dissection. There are essentially two types of resectoscopes, which differ in outer diameter: (1) 7.3 mm (22 Fr); (2) 8.7 mm (26 Fr). The 8.7 mm-resectoscope is commonly used only in patients with a large uterus (endometrial ablation) or in the presence of pathologies (myoma) with a diameter larger than 3 cm, or if a myoma is found to have a difficult intramural location. In cases which require dilation of the cervical canal (Hegar no. 8), the 22-Fr resectoscope is usually preferred. The resectoscope consists of a classic endoscope, with diameters ranging between 2.9 mm and 4 mm, preferably with a 12° viewing angle to keep the electrode within the field of view, combined with a cutting loop operated by a passive spring mechanism, and two sheaths for continuous irrigation and suction of the distension medium. Apart from the cutting loop, other instruments such as micro knives and a variety of vaporizing or coagulating electrodes can be used with the working element of the resectoscope. All these instruments are available for both the 22-Fr and the 26-Fr resectoscope. The same resectoscope can be used both as unipolar and bipolar instrument, simply by changing the working element and the electrodes. For distension and irrigation of the uterine cavity, a 1.5% glycine solution or sorbitol mannitol is used, as previously stated, for unipolar surgery. For bipolar resectoscopy, physiological saline solution must be used as distension medium.[1,5]

Surgical instruments are available in both rigid and flexible forms to be inserted through the operating channels of the scopes. Examples of surgical instruments and their uses are listed below (Figs. 6 and 7):

- Scissors: To incise a septum, excise a polyp, or lyse synechiae
- Biopsy forceps: To perform directed biopsy for pathologic review
- Grasping instruments: To remove foreign bodies
- Roller ball, barrel, or ellipsoid: To perform endometrial ablation and/or desiccation (This instrument is used with a resectoscope)
- Loop electrode: To resect a fibroid or polyp or endometrium (This instrument is used with a resectoscope)
- Scalpel: To cut or coagulate tissue, with high power density at its tip (This instrument is used with a resectoscope)
- Vaporizing electrodes: To destroy endometrial polyps, fibroids, intrauterine adhesions, and septa; also used for endometrial ablation (This instrument is used with a resectoscope)
- Morcellator: To cut and remove endometrial polyps or fibroids.[4]

Improvements in hysteroscope design have improved the effectiveness of the inflow-outflow channels and of specific operating instruments. For example, the Chip E-Vac System (Richard Wolf Medical Instruments Corporation, Vernon Hill, IL) incorporates a suction channel and a pump to aid in removing chips of tissue during resection. This feature improves visibility and may decrease time otherwise spent emptying the pieces from the endometrial cavity. Another instrument in the forefront is a hysteroscopic morcellator (Smith & Nephew, Inc., Andover, Mass), which may reduce myomectomy and polypectomy time by morcellating and removing tissue in

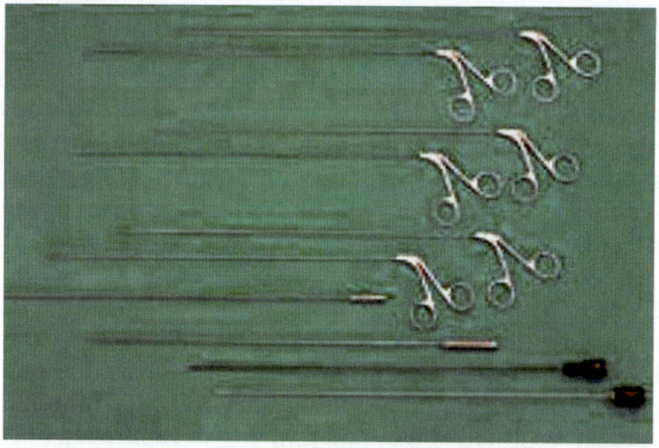

Fig. 6: Instruments that can be inserted through the office hysteroscope: forceps, scissors, unipolar and bipolar electrodes.

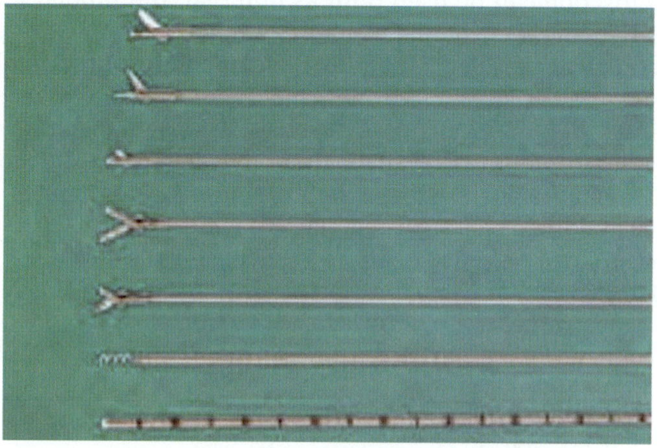

Fig. 7: Semi-rigid instruments: forceps, biopsy forceps, scissors and myoma fixation instrument.

one movement under direct visualization. It requires cervical dilation to 9 mm. A new hysteroscopic morcellating system called MyoSure (Interlace Medical, Inc., Framingham, Mass) is reported to work just as well, removing submucosal fibroids up to 3 cm in diameter, with a unit that only requires cervical dilation to 6 mm. This smaller diameter suggests it may be used in an office setting.[4]

ELECTROSURGICAL UNIT FOR HIGH-FREQUENCY SURGERY

The resectoscope is connected to a high-frequency electrosurgical unit with automatic power supply control and alarm function. Modern high-frequency systems can be operated both in unipolar and bipolar mode, for hysteroscopy as well as for laparoscopy and open surgery. Resectoscopy can be performed with unipolar or bipolar current depending on the available system. In the unipolar system, the electrons flow from the high-frequency electrosurgical unit to the active electrode (e.g. cutting loop or knife electrode) before passing through the tissue to the neutral electrode and then returning to the electrosurgical unit. In the bipolar system, the high-frequency generator produces an initial peak of around 400 RMSV (root mean square voltage) which creates an electrical arc between the two bipolar electrodes. Once the electrode is sufficiently close to the tissue, the electrical arc converts the conductive solution of sodium chloride to a plasma containing sodium particles that are active because they are highly charged with energy. Once this plasma effect has been created, it can be maintained with a lower voltage (100–350 RMSV). Contact with the activated sodium ions (and thus not with the electrode) provokes disintegration of the tissue due to breaking of the carbon-carbon and carbon-hydrogen bonds and dissociation of the water molecules to H+ and hydroxide ion (OH-) ions. The result is collapse of the cellular membranes with ensuing cutting of the tissue.

The temperature of the surrounding tissues remains between 40° and 70° using the bipolar system but reaches 400° when the unipolar system is used resulting in deep surrounding tissue changes.[1,7] Electrosurgery can be used for coagulation, dissection and also for combination of both modes using nonmodulated (soft coagulation) and modulated flow (spray coagulation). The coagulation current is characterized by intermittent phases of electrical activity which cause dehydration of the cells and coagulation of the proteins with successive hemostasis. The nonmodulated cutting current is a continuous flow of electrons which produces a rapid increase of temperature inside the cells causing them to explode. Use of nonmodulated current is recommended for coagulation as lower voltages current is used. It is a less risky option and as efficacious as the modulated coagulation current[6] (Fig. 8).

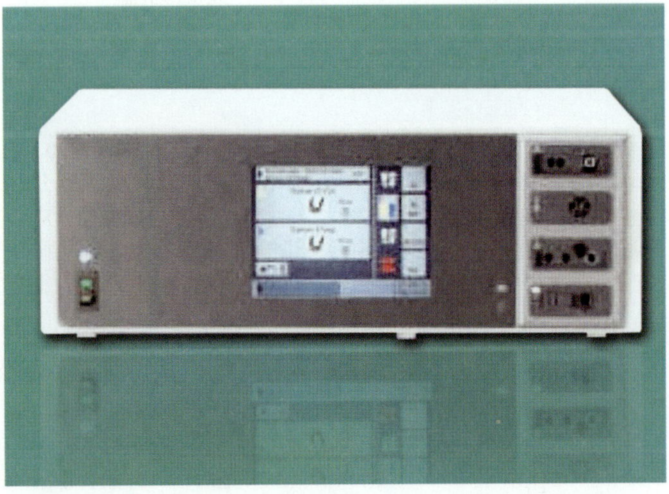

Fig. 8: High-frequency electrosurgical unit AUTOCON@II 400.

HYSTEROSCOPIC LASER SURGERY

Argon, neodymium, YAG and KTP lasers are the most frequently used lasers in hysteroscopy and have good characteristics in terms of coagulation, although they do have some weak points in terms of vaporization. Laser generators are significantly more expensive than electrosurgical equipment and do not offer particular advantages in clinical practice.[1]

MAINTENANCE AND STERILIZATION OF INSTRUMENTS

Autoclave sterilization is the cheapest system, and owing to the diffusion of steam, it cleans even the smallest gaps and openings. Only the optical systems and instruments which are specifically certified for the autoclave may be sterilized with a 20-minute cycle at 121°C or 7 minutes at 134°C.

Gas sterilization with ethylene oxide is an ideal system since it is performed at low temperatures obviating the risk of damaging the endoscopic instruments.[8]

REFERENCES

1. Mencaglia L, De Albuquerque Neto LC, Alfonso Arias Alvarez R. Manual of Hysteroscopy: Diagnostic, Operative and Office Hysteroscopy. Tuttlingen: End Press; 2014.
2. Litta P, Bonora M, Pozzan C, et al. Carbon dioxide versus normal saline in outpatient hysteroscopy. Hum Reprod. 2003;18(11):2446-9.
3. Valle RF, Sciarra JJ. Current status of hysteroscopy in gynaecological practice. Fertil Steril. 1979;32:619-32.
4. Petrozza JC, Attaman JA. Hysteroscopy. Drug Dis Obs Gyn. 2015.
5. Bettocchi S1, Nappi L, Ceci O, et al. What does diagnostic hysteroscopy mean today? The role of the new techniques. Curr Opin Obstet Gynecol. 2003;15(4):303-8.
6. Di Spiezio Sardo A, Taylor A, Tsirkas P, et al. Hysteroscopy: a technique for all? Analysis of 5,000 outpatient hysteroscopies. 2008;89:438-43.
7. Ozturk E1, Ugur MG, Balat O, et al. An analysis of hysteroscopy experience over a seven year period. Clin Exp Obstet Gynecol. 2010;37(2):150-1.
8. Block SS. Disinfection, Sterilization, and Preservation in Hospitals, 5th edition. Philadelphia: Lippincott Williams & Wilkins; 2001.

Chapter 2

Ideal Anesthesia for Hysteroscopy

Nibedita Pani, Srimanta Haldar

BACKGROUND

Use of the hysteroscope in modern gynecological practice continues to develop as a diagnostic and management tool for intrauterine disease. Operative hysteroscopy (OH) is now an accepted alternative to hysterectomy for women with menorrhagia. The advantages of OH are associated with its short operating time, rapid postoperative recovery and low morbidity. However, there are concerns about the potential serious complications which can occur during and following OH, and it is important that both surgeons and anesthetists are aware of these—especially as many procedures take place as day-cases.

ANESTHETIC CONSIDERATIONS

- Fluid overload leading to hyponatremia and hypo-osmolality
- Glycine toxicity
- Hemorrhage
- Hypothermia
- Uterine perforation
- Gas or air embolism
- Patient positioning to prevent peripheral neuropathy
- Prevention of sepsis.

CHOICE OF ANESTHESIA

The type of anesthesia used depends on the procedure, the patient's level of anxiety, the surgeon and anesthesiologist's expertise. Simple diagnostic procedures can be completed with monitored anesthesia care with paracervical block or intrauterine local anesthesia. But for extensive procedures or for patients with a low pain tolerance or electrosurgery, general anesthesia (GA) or regional anesthesia is indicated to ensure that the patient does not move with uterine stimulation to avoid the risk uterine perforation and intraperitoneal injury.

PREANESTHETIC ASSESSMENT

History and Examination

Cardiovascular: Hypertension, ischemic heart disease (IHD) and arrhythmias (particularly atrial fibrillation) are common. Patients with recent onset or poorly controlled heart failure have the highest perioperative mortality.

Respiratory: Marked decrease in functional ability (e.g. inability to climb one flight of stairs) suggests severe disease. Inability to lie flat because of dyspnea from cardiac or respiratory causes will make awake regional anesthesia poorly tolerated.

Neurological: Confused patients may be not lie still during spinal anesthesia.

Musculoskeletal: Degenerative changes in the vertebral column may make subarachnoid block (SAB) technically difficult. Arthritic joints or joint replacements are susceptible to damage or dislocation when the patient's legs are placed in the lithotomy position for the procedure.

Renal impairment if present may deteriorate due to fluid overload.

Airway: Even if SAB is planned perform a full anesthetic assessment (e.g. anticipated airway difficulties) in case the regional technique fails or is inadequate.

Investigations: Full blood count or hemoglobin level, blood glucose, electrolytes and creatinine and electrocardiogram (ECG). Chest X-ray (CXR) if indicated.

GENERAL ANESTHESIA

Advantages

The advantages of GA are:

- Patients with chest disease may not tolerate lying flat or be able to suppress their cough
- No time constraints. Suitable for lengthy procedures
- May be less hemodynamically challenging than SAB in patients with cardiac problems such as aortic stenosis (and other fixed output states) and IHD
- Allows better control of CO_2, which may reduce bleeding from the uterine bed
- Preferred for patients with low pain tolerance and anxiety
- Preferred for extensive surgeries and when concurrent laparoscopy is to be performed.

Risks

Lithotomy, head-down reduces tidal volume (Vt) and functional residual capacity (FRC). Position also increases the risk of aspiration. Under light planes of GA, uterine stimulation can interfere with surgery—this can be managed by deepening anesthesia. Postoperative analgesia will be needed.

REGIONAL ANESTHESIA

The advantages of the regional technique include:

- Early detection of complications such as fluid overload and uterine perforation
- Possible reduced blood loss, requiring fewer transfusions
- Avoids effects of GA on pulmonary pathology
- Good early postoperative analgesia
- Reduced incidence of postoperative deep venous thrombosis (DVT)/ pulmonary embolism (PE)
- Lower cost.

SPINAL ANESTHESIA

Low spinal anesthesia (with or without intrathecal opioid) achieving a block up to T10 level for the management of patients undergoing OH may offer, in addition to a reliable block and stable hemodynamics, less operative cognitive impairment, a low incidence of side effects, good intraoperative and postoperative analgesia, and acceptable patient satisfaction without prolonging recovery room discharge.

PARACERVICAL BLOCK

Innervation of the uterus and cervix is complex. Major autonomic nerves arise from the S2 to S4 roots and travel to the uterus in the lower portion of the broad ligament as the Frankenhäuser plexus. Interruption of this plexus is the basis of the paracervical block. However, the uterus is richly innervated with nerves that originate at other points as well. Alternative methods of local anesthesia targeting other nerve plexuses may improve pain management in procedures.

Common anesthetic agents are 1% lidocaine, mepivacaine, prilocaine, ropivacaine, bupivacaine, and etidocaine. Of these, bupivacaine and etidocaine have longer durations and can last upward of 2–3 hours.

A recent study suggests that paracervical ropivacaine controls intraoperative pain slightly better than lidocaine during surgical abortions. In most cases, 10 mL of bupivacaine 0.25%, mepivacaine 1%, or lidocaine 1–2% is an adequate volume for paracervical anesthesia.

Risks

Bradycardia and hypotension.

INTRAUTERINE ANESTHESIA

The effectiveness of intrauterine anesthetic is related to the origin and pathways of uterine innervation. While the Frankenhäuser plexus in the lower broad ligament is the most well-known nervous pathway, the uterus, cervix and

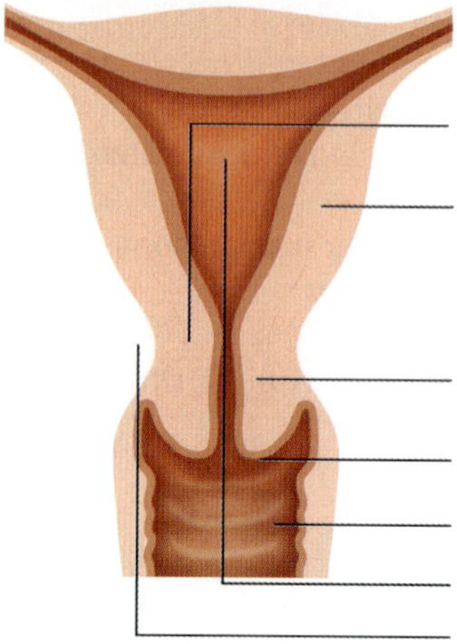

Fig. 1: Different methods of administration of local anesthetic for outpatient hysteroscopy.

fallopian tubes receive nerve supply from other sources as well. Sympathetic innervations from the T10 to L1 roots enter the uterus with the utero-ovarian vessels and follow a variable course, with branches following the anastomoses of the uterine artery. Well-defined nerve plexuses lie in the endometrium and along the mucosal surface of the cervix, and are fed by both the ascending and descending roots; the precise pattern of innervation varies with pathologic processes such as endometriosis and adenomyosis. The limited efficacy of the paracervical block in many gynecologic procedures is likely due to its inability to block these nerves of other origins. Intrauterine anesthesia may reach these nerves more effectively and, alone or in conjunction with paracervical block, provide more global uterine anesthesia (Fig. 1).

Advantages

Administering intrauterine anesthesia prior to an office procedure is an effective, low-cost, and low-risk intervention. Administration is generally simple, and seems less painful for patients than injection of a paracervical block. Good effect on pain is most consistently seen with doses at or equivalent to 100–200 mg of lidocaine.

Risks

Inadequate anesthesia and local anesthesia toxicity.

POSTOPERATIVE COMPLICATIONS

Hypothermia, hypotension, hemorrhage, septicemia and signs and symptoms of fluid overload can all present in the recovery room. Patients may become acutely hypotensive after lowering their legs from the lithotomy position because the reduction in venous return. Severe, persistent or unexpected pelvic/abdominal pain, heavy vaginal bleeding and hypotension indicate uterine perforation. The symptoms of this may be masked by residual SAB.

CONCLUSION

Today, the ideal anesthesia for outpatient hysteroscopy is still being sought. However, it appears that the use of combined local intracervical and direct intrauterine anesthesia is effective for office hysteroscopy while GA/regional anesthesia is still the preferred technique for extensive hysteroscopic procedures.

BIBLIOGRAPHY

1. Agdi M, Tulandi T. Outpatient hysteroscopy with combined local intracervical and intrauterine anesthesia. Gynecol Obstet Invest. 2010;69:30-2.
2. Mercier RJ, Zerden ML. Intrauterine anesthesia for gynecologic procedures: a systematic review. Obstet Gynecol. 2012;120(3):669-77.
3. Murdoch JA, Gan TJ. Anesthesia for hysteroscopy. Anesthesiol Clin North America. 2001;19(1):125-40.
4. Mushambi MC, Williamson K. Anaesthetic considerations for hysteroscopic surgery. Best Pract Res Clin Anaesthesiol. 2002;16(1):35-52.

Chapter 3

Basic Principles in Operative Hysteroscopy

S Krishnakumar, Rohan Krishnakumar

INTRODUCTION

Hysteroscopy has revolutionized the diagnosis and management of intrauterine pathologies and today operative hysteroscopy is considered, in majority, a continuation of diagnostic hysteroscopy.

The revolutionary changes in instrumentation and techniques have helped in classifying surgical hysteroscopy as:

1. *Operative hysteroscopy:* Those done with smaller diameter operative sheath without much use of electrical energy. This can apply to 75% of surgical pathologies.
2. *Resectoscopic surgery:* Those, where the resectoscope and electrical energy are used.

Though at many centers in different parts of the world, operative hysteroscopic surgeries with operative hysteroscopic sheath are being done in outpatient settings without anesthesia and the Resectoscopic surgeries requiring anesthesia are performed in full operating room (OR) settings, I would opine that our country and patient profile is still not ready for this, though our center uses office hysteroscopy in at least 20% of hysteroscopic procedures.

CONTRAINDICATIONS FOR OPERATIVE HYSTEROSCOPIC SURGERY (ABSOLUTE AND RELATIVE)

- Pelvic inflammatory disease
- Acute cervicovaginitis
- Severe metrorrhagia
- Pregnancy
- Inappropriate instrumentation and technology
- Inadequate surgical skill and experience.

Preoperative Requisites

1. Complete standard blood investigations (preoperative) and electrolytes if glycine is to be used.

2. Electrocardiography (ECG) and echo should be done in obese and elderly patients.
3. Proper imaging: Good transvaginal sonography is a must, hysterosalpingography in selected cases.
4. Surgery should be always done in immediate postmenstrual phase.
5. Bladder should be empty.
6. Good motorized table with lithotomy arrangements (Allen stirrups if available and patient's buttocks should be just outside the edge of the table. The surgeons chair should have wheels for easy movement (Fig. 1).
7. Availability of good endoscopic camera with monitor, light source [Xenon/light-emitting diode (LED)], Hysteromat, electric generator (Fig. 2) with bipolar energy capabilities, and full set of operative hysteroscopic and resectoscopic instruments.

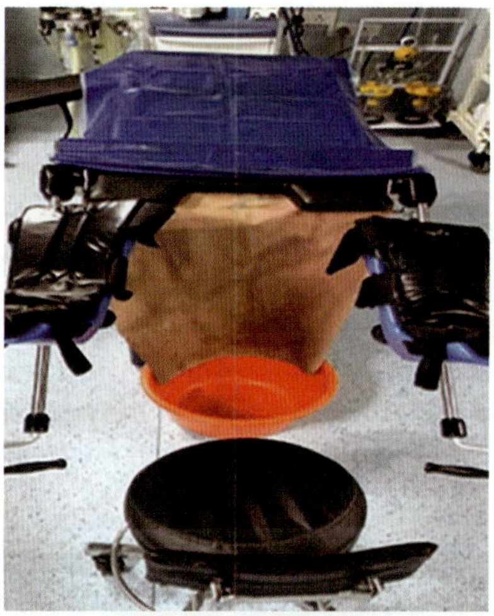

Fig. 1: Allen stirrups.

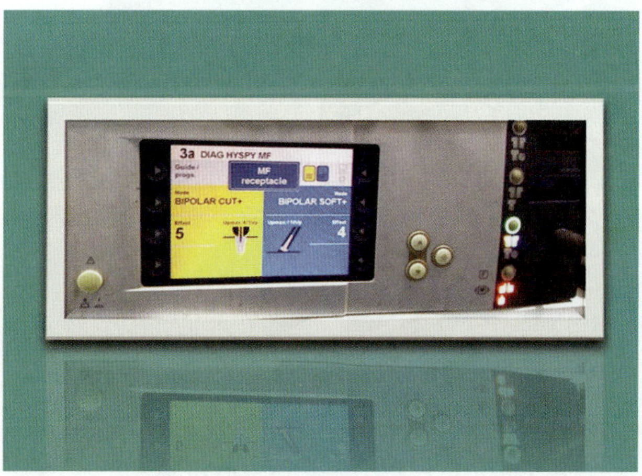

Fig. 2: Hysteromat.

8. *Anesthesia:* Though epidural anesthesia is best as the patient is conscious to inform of any untoward side effects, in majority of the case we prefer general anesthesia with full multipara monitoring.
9. *Counseling:* Regarding type of surgery, limitations, complications, and 2 stage procedures in selected cases (large submucus myomas and severe Asherman's syndrome).

OPERATIVE HYSTEROSCOPY

Instrumentation

With all the advantages of no touch vaginoscopic method, standard 2.9 mm 30° telescope with a 5 mm oval shaped operative sheath with inflow and outflow channels an channel to introduce 2 mm operative instruments (Fig. 3), which may include various biopsy forceps, graspers, scissors (Fig. 4), and electrodes (Fig. 5). Sterile inflow and outflow tube is a must for proper distension. We prefer the double ended washer (Fig. 6) to prevent leaking of distension media. All the required instruments should be readily available (Fig. 7).

Distension Media and Delivery

With patient safety, at operative hysteroscopy being the prime criteria, normal saline (Table 1) should be the media of choice and delivery system should be good operative pump (Fig. 8A), capable of delivering the media at correct inflow per minute and measuring the correct intrauterine pressure at every stage of the procedure. EASI hysteromat (Fig. 8B) is one such new device with settings

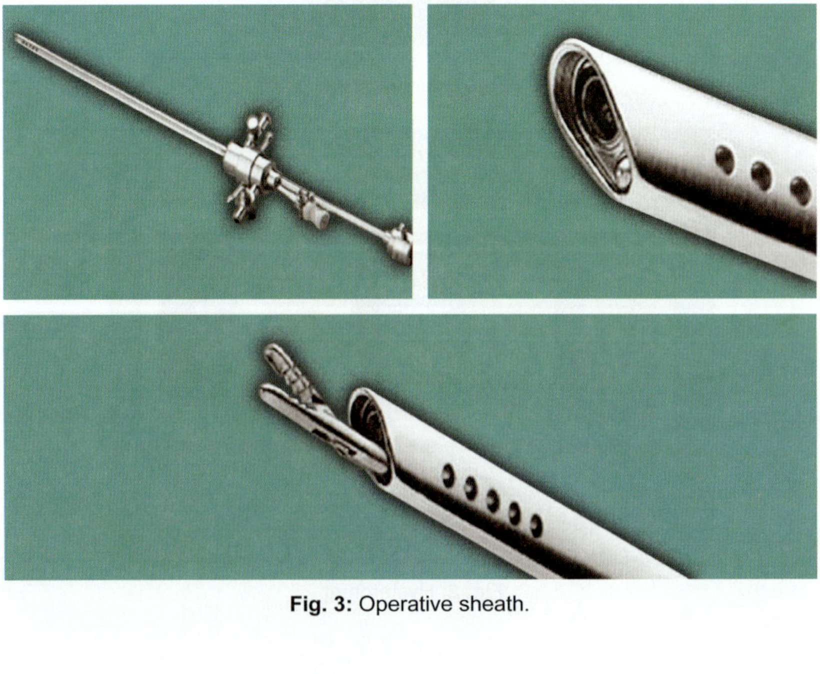

Fig. 3: Operative sheath.

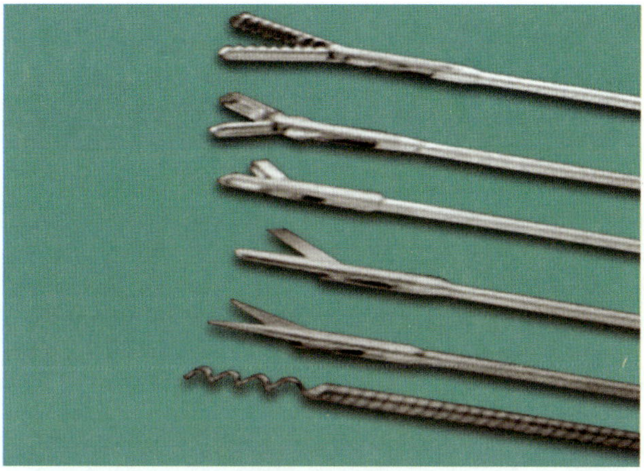

Fig. 4: Scissors.

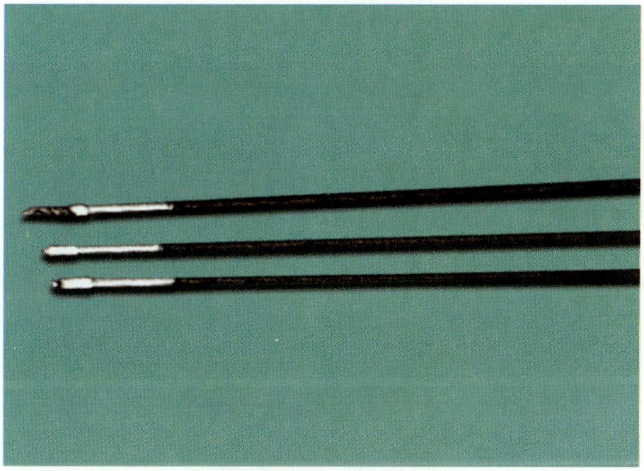

Fig. 5: Electrodes.

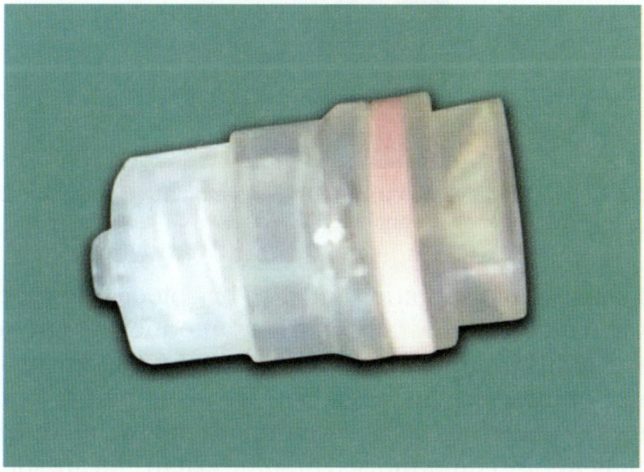

Fig. 6: Double ended washer.

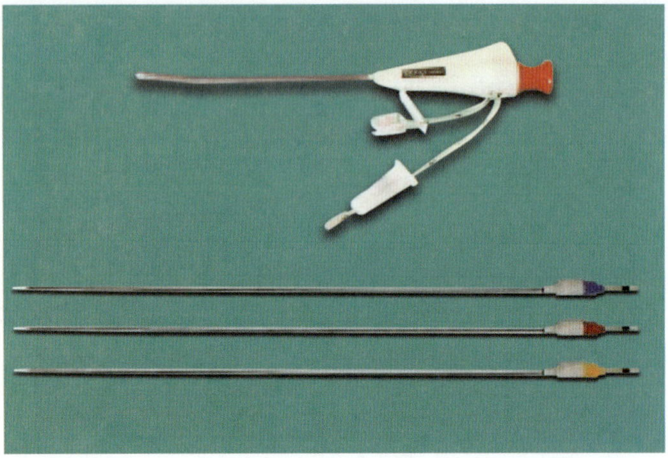

Fig. 7: Important instruments for vaginoscopic method.

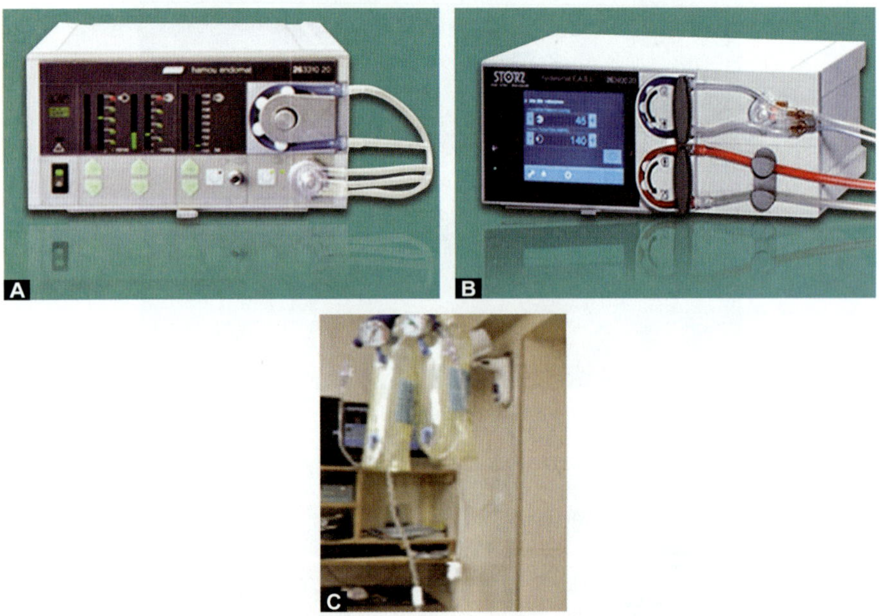

Figs. 8A to C: (A) Operative pump. (B) EASI hysteromat. (C) Pressure bags with connected TUR set.

for different sheaths and surgeries and also has blood and mucus mode to remove debris at different flow rates, with intrauterine pressure settings from 45 mmHg to 75 mmHg. It also has proper outflow measurement of fluid used. In the absence of these expensive gadgets we recommend, 2 pressure bags with connected TUR set (Fig. 8C) for continuous inflow, but the pressure and flow measurements are compromised to some extent, but are still satisfactory if the surgical time is not prolonged.

Table 1: Electrolyte content and osmolality of hysteroscopic distending solutions.

Solution	*Na mEq/L*	*Cl mEq/L*	*mOsm/L*
0.9% Sodium chloride	154	154	308
Lactated Ringers	130	110	275
0.45% Sodium chloride	77	77	155
3% Sorbitol	–	–	178
1.5% Glycine	–	–	200
5% Mannitol	–	–	275
5% Dextrose in water	–	–	250

But it is mandatory that an assistant is dedicated to measure the fluid deficit and the outflow fluid also be strictly measured. We prefer to also use underpad, as shown in Figure 9, to collect all the fluid that leaks out of the cervix and vagina.

Today, with availability of good bipolar saline of glycine is to be avoided in all cases. The surgery should be stopped once the fluid deficit crosses, 1,500 mL in case of glycine and in case of saline 2,000 mL deficit can still be managed.

Standard Principles in Operative Hysteroscopy

1. Tubal ostia are always the landmark for safe surgery and fundus is always a little lower than ostia.

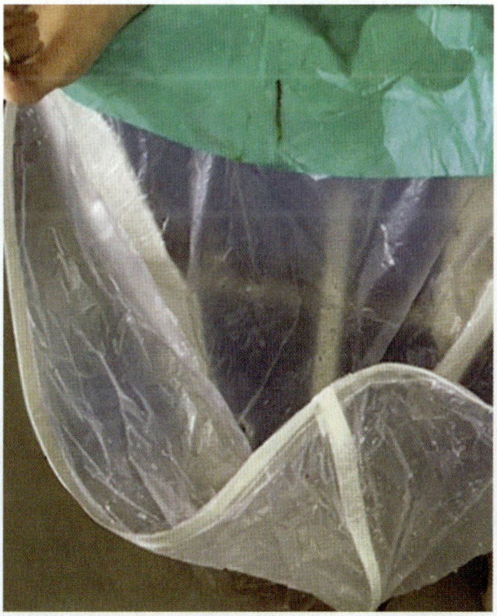

Fig. 9: Underpad to collect all the fluid that leaks out of the cervix and vagina.

2. Orientation of normal hysteroscopic anatomy comes with experience and one must do sufficient diagnostic hysteroscopy before embarking upon operative hysteroscopy.
3. Endometrium is a very delicate tender epithelium and use of electrosurgery may hamper proper endometrial growth especially in reproductive age group and always one should prefer to use mechanical energy in cases of infertility hysteroscopic surgery. There are no studies recommending one over the other.
4. Monitor and maintain all the safety recommendations on fluid deficit and intrauterine pressure.
5. When removing tissues after biopsy or foreign bodies remove the whole system in toto as the tissue or foreign body will not enter the instrument channel and will slip out of the grasper.

Indications

1. Abnormal and postmenopausal bleeding-targeted biopsy. To get a good quantity of tissue push the grasper into the endometrium or cut with scissors for adequate biopsy.
2. Removal of foreign bodies/retained products of conception (RPOC).
3. *Septum:* All case of septum should be attempted to cut with scissors and only in very large septum with broad base and those with more fibromuscular tissue we use resectoscope. Always begin cutting at the apex of the inverted triangle (Fig. 10) and keeping the ostia as the landmark midline is maintained and in case of very tough tissues or excess vascularity change over to resectoscope with bipolar energy. Always spare scissors should be available for good complete surgical outcome. Always stop cutting once the normal anatomy is restored (ostia is always just above the

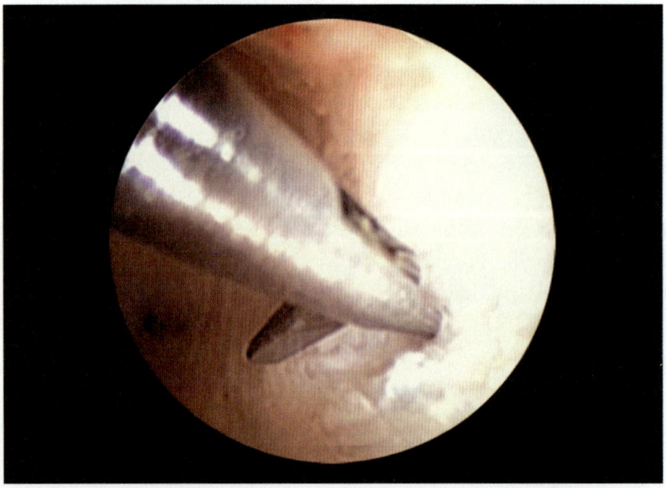

Fig. 10: Technique to dissect septum (inverted triangle).

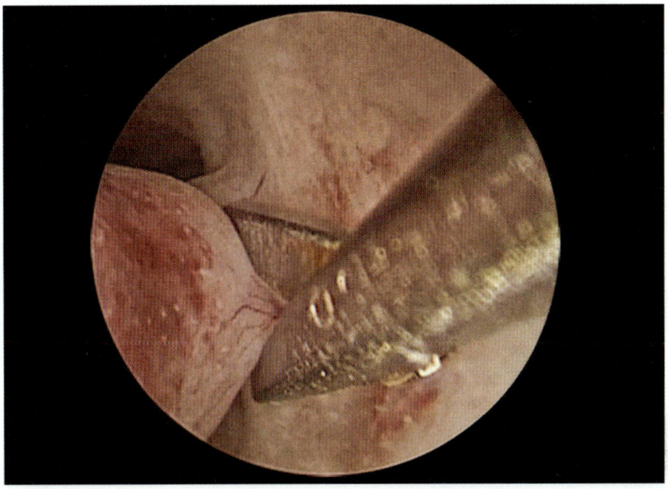

Fig. 11: Removal of polyps.

fundus). Use of laparoscope is restricted to patients with doubtful didelphys uterus only.

4. *Polyps:* Polyps up to 2 cm can be safely removed with operative channel instruments. The polyp may be required to be sliced with scissors in to smaller pieces (Fig. 11) and removed with graspers. Occasionally for vascular polyps, bipolar needle can be used to slice and reduce bleeding.
5. *Intrauterine adhesions:* In every case of suspected Asherman's syndrome, it is ideal to use smaller diameter operative sheath only as anatomy is distorted at the beginning and any dilation with its disadvantages of blood, false passage, etc. will make the entry in to uterine cavity more difficult and messy. We always prefer to insert scissors in the operative channel at the beginning only as if there are adhesions at the cervical canal or internal os they can be cut for entry under vision (Fig. 12). The cervical mucosal fold is the landmark for correct entry in to the endometrial cavity as folds from all sides of cervical canal will meet at internal os only, and in case of total Asherman's syndrome it is the only landmark to enter the correct plane. At many stages mere opening of the blades of scissors will give way to the correct plane and cutting with scissors may be restricted to very fibrous tissues. Though ostia is a landmark in all hysteroscopic surgeries, one may not be able to locate the same in severe Asherman's syndrome and one need not go on cutting to see the ostia. Surgery is considered optimum if adequate endometrial size and shape is achieved.

Resectoscopic Surgery

With all the advantages of vaginoscopic method of performing hysteroscopic surgery the use of resectoscope is restricted to the following indications:

- Large, or multiple or vascular polyps
- Submucus myomas

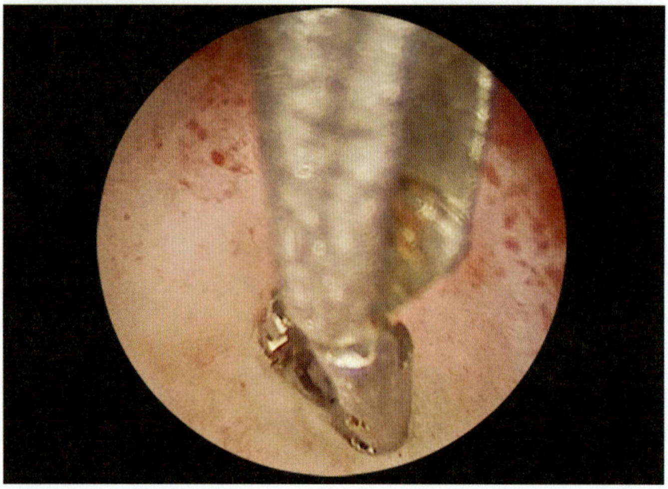

Fig. 12: Removal of intrauterine adhesions.

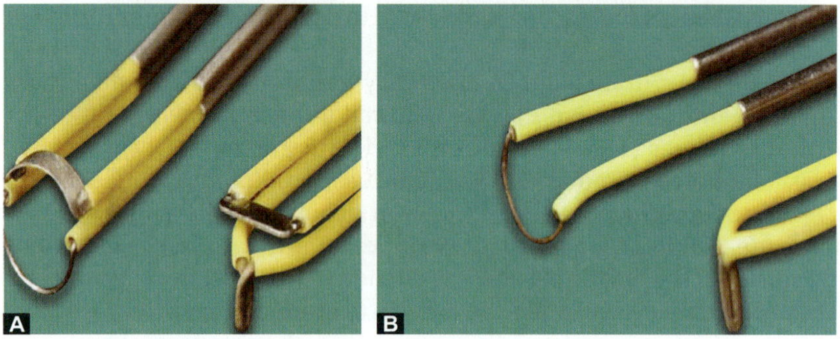

Figs. 13A and B: (A) Bipolar current. (B) Monopolar current.

- Very large broad based fleshy septum
- Endometrial resection.

Principles for Safe Resectoscopic Surgery

1. 24–26 Fr diameter resectoscope is better as the tissue resection is bigger and allows for faster surgery as duration of surgery is of prime importance to limit fluid deficit.
2. Bipolar current (Fig. 13A) is better than monopolar (Fig. 13B) as distension media is saline and avoids all the ill effects of glycine overload.
3. Always use the current only if vision is adequate.
4. Begin resection from above downwards and never below upwards.
5. Step on the pedal before touching the tissue and take care the adjacent healthy endometrium is less touched with current (Fig. 14).
6. Restrict removal of the resectoscope out of the uterine cavity as every insertion will waste more time to remove blood and debris.

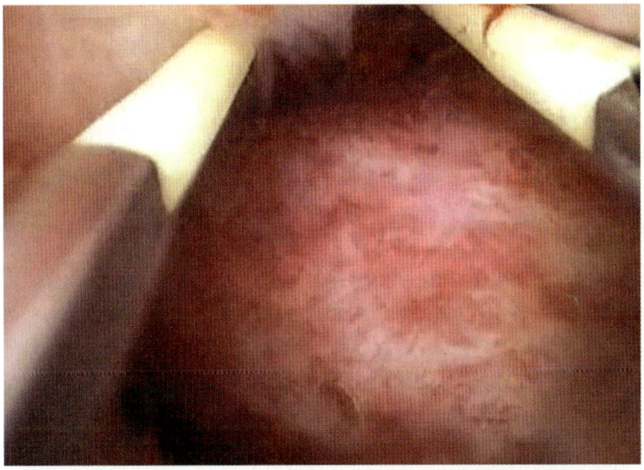

Fig. 14: Removal of endometrial polyp.

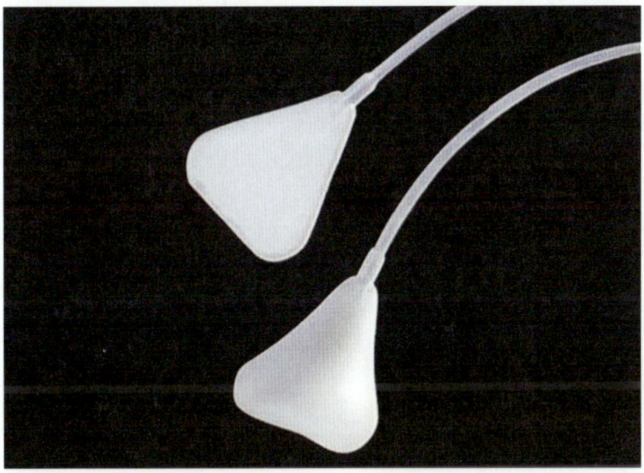

Fig. 15: Intrauterine balloon.

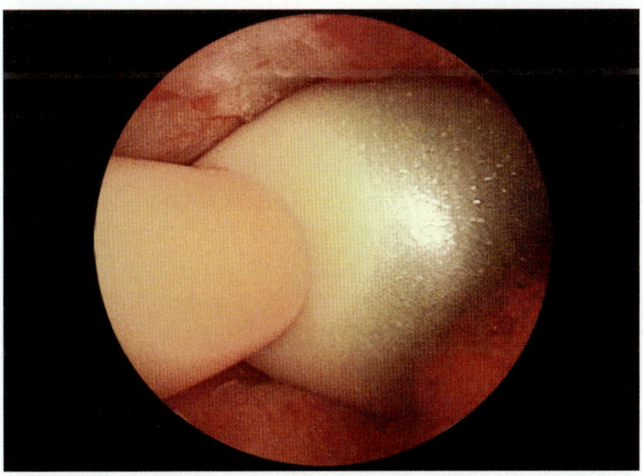

Fig. 16: Pediatric Foley catheter.

7. Push the resected tissues to the upper part of cavity and away from the area of surgery.
8. Stop the surgery in the event of improper vision, sudden collapse of the distension crossing of the recommended fluid deficit. Always complicated surgery can be completed at a second setting.

Prevention of Adhesions and Recurrences of Adhesions

Though there is no randomized control studies to recommend the best step to prevent adhesions, the following standard steps are followed after major operative hysteroscopy to prevent adhesions.

- Intrauterine balloon (Fig. 15) or pediatric Foley catheter (Fig. 16).
- Estrogen supplements for at least two cycles.
- Adhesion barriers like hyaluronidase have been proven beneficial in certain studies.
- Always relook hysteroscopy is to be done especially in all cases of infertility especially if electric energy is used and in cases of severe Asherman's syndrome and large septum.

It is highly recommended to follow the safety recommendations to master hysteroscopic surgery.

Chapter 4

Microhysteroscopy, Contact Hysteroscopy and Office Hysteroscopy

Sujata Swain

INTRODUCTION

Hysteroscopy procedure has now become the gold standard for diagnosis of intrauterine pathology. Modern hysteroscopy has attained various facets to it. It has widened its arms to incorporate various diagnostic and therapeutic procedures, and also, it has tried to increase the ease of the procedure, patient compliance and decrease the treatment span. Microhysteroscopy, contact hysteroscopy, and office hysteroscopy have made the procedure more complaint and have also immensely increased its avenue as a diagnostic and therapeutic tool.

MICROHYSTEROSCOPY

The microhysteroscope was developed by Hamou[1,2] in France in 1979 and has been approved for use in the United States since 1981. The recently developed microhysteroscope, which offers a combination of panoramic hysteroscopy, contact hysteroscopy, and microhysteroscopy. Aspects that are common to other hysteroscopic techniques include timing, clinical history, positioning of the patient, physical examination, Pap smear, and ruling of pregnancy or infection.

Technique

The light source does not vary from that used in conventional hysteroscopy, but the uterine cavity is distended with CO_2 gas, which should be delivered with a specific hysteroflator at a rate of no more than 100 mL/min (30–70 mL/min) and a maximum intrauterine pressure of 90 mmHg.

The sheath encasing the endoscope is 5 mm in diameter and usually can be introduced without dilatation. Anesthesia may not be required. Because of the size of the endoscope, the endocervix is crossed under direct vision, taking advantage of the CO_2 microcavity created in front of the distal end of the endoscope. The endocervix is observed at 20X magnification. Once the internal

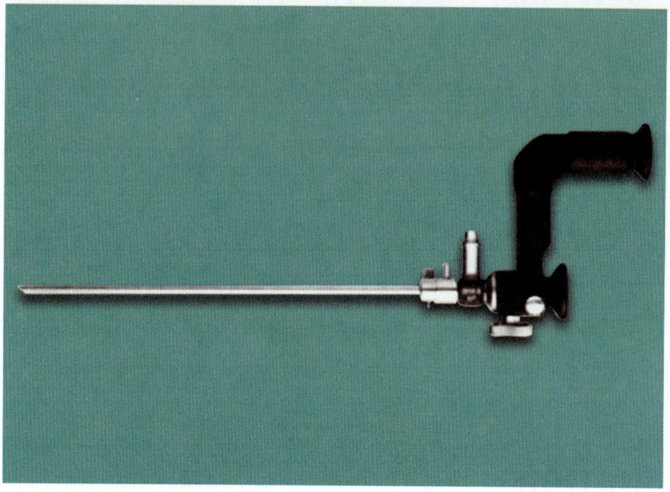

Fig. 1: Contact microcolpohysteroscope with a double ocular. The 30° for oblique, 4 mm outer diameter (OD) telescope is encased in a 5 mm OD sheath.
Sourec: K Storz

cervical os is crossed and the endoscope provides a view of the uterine cavity, the microhysteroscope is reset at unit magnification, and panoramic viewing of the cavity can begin. For detailed observation of any specific area within the cavity, the instrument can be set at 20X magnification; this is particularly helpful in visualizing the uterotubal cones and the first millimeter of the tubal openings. (Fig. 1)

The size of the endoscope also permits examination of the area of the endometrium indented by the distal portion of the instrument and assessment of its thickness.[2,3]

Applications

The diagnostic applications are the same as for conventional hysteroscopy. The main advantage of this endoscope is that it frees intrauterine adhesions by pressing with the sharp edge of its biangulated end, allowing target abrasions of the adhesions.[4,5]

It has been used in the evaluation of endometrial morphology, with special attention to the evaluation of blood vessels and endometrial gland openings. These evaluations are performed on contact, utilizing magnifications at 60X–80X, and occasionally 150X.

Van Herendael[6] and associates reported on the microhysteroscopic evaluation of the endometrium for endometrial dating. Although this attempt cannot replace histopathologic examination, it has helped to understand the physiologic changes that the endometrium undergoes during each phase of the cycle (Table 1) (Fig. 2).

Bettocchi[3] and colleagues described abnormal vascular patterns, different from those discovered during normal cyclicity, in patient with abnormal

Table 1: Physiologic changes in endometrium during each phase of the menstrual cycle.

	Menstrual	*Proliferative*	*Early luteal*	*Late luteal*
Days	1–4	5–14	14–21	22–28
Color	Red	Pink	White	White
Surface	Irregular	Smooth	Wavy	Spongy
Thickness	0–1 mm	2–5 mm	>6 mm	>7 mm
Glands	Absent	White dots	Prominent	Absent
Notch	No	Hemorrhagic	Serous	Serous
Vessels	No	Thin vessels	Absent	Absent

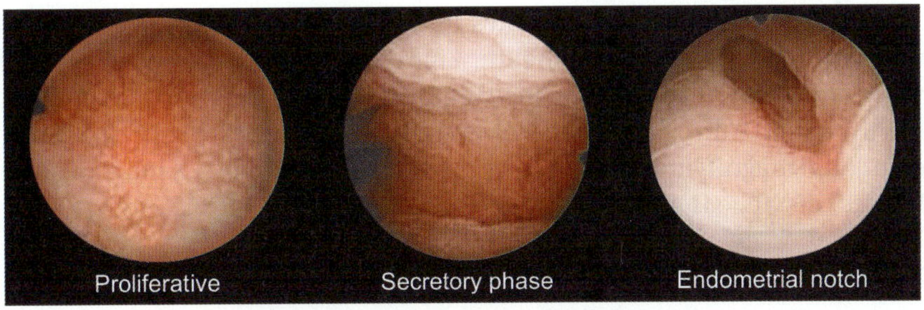

Fig. 2: Phases of menstrual cycle.

uterine bleeding who nonetheless had an apparently normal view on panoramic hysteroscopic examination.

Other applications are in embryoscopy and salpingoscopy; the endoscope can be introduced atraumatically to visualize the early embryo through a chorionic window. An application of the endoscope is placement of intratubal devices as an ambulatory procedure.[7]

It can also be used as microhysteroscope. Abnormalities such as leukoplakia, mosaicism, punctation, or colpitis then become apparent. The cervix is systematically inspected and the transformation zone explored. Because the instrument is in contact with the mucosa, there is automatic focusing. This ensures proper biopsy and treatment.

The diagnosis of dysplasia depends on the observation of severe nuclear abnormalities in the regularity of cells in the same optical field. These abnormalities include irregularity, hyperchromasia, and especially nuclei in excess of 15 mm associated with anisokaryosis and dyskaryosis, with nucleocytoplasmic dysmaturation and marked mitotic activity.

A comparison study of microhysteroscopy and colposcopy, cytology suggest that microhysteroscopy is a precise method for evaluating cervical intraepithelial neoplasia (CIN), thus permitting detailed microscopic evaluation in vivo. It plays a complementary role in cytology, colposcopy, and histologic evaluation of CIN.

CONTACT HYSTEROSCOPY (FIG. 3)

Contact hysteroscopy is an endoscopic technique that enables visualization of the uterine interior without distension of the uterine cavity, as is required with conventional hysteroscopy. In addition, the contact hysteroscope is free of external electrical connections and simply requires ambient light.

From a historic perspective, the instrument used currently has evolved from a concept originally introduced by David[8] in 1907. For past 10 years, it has been popularized by Parent[9] and associates and Barbot[10] in Europe, and by Baggish in the United States.

Instrumentation

It consists of a light collector that gathers and transmits ambient light down a rod of optical glass that terminates in a mirror-type lens. The glass rod is enclosed in a stainless steel sheath. Light is transmitted and reflected by internal mirrors and lenses. The instrument is 200 mm long and is available in both 6 mm and 8 mm diameters. The eyepiece magnification is 1.6X, although an optional magnifying device allows the user an additional 2X magnification. The focal distance is 4 mm or less.

Technique

It can be performed by local paracervical anesthesia or under general anesthesia, if other surgical procedures are contemplated. In many cases, a multiparous uterus requires little or no cervical dilatation, and the 6 mm instrumentation is sufficient. Because of the short focal distance,

Illumination	Inspection
Natural or artificial (outside light projector, skylight)	Visual
Flash projector	Photography cinematography television

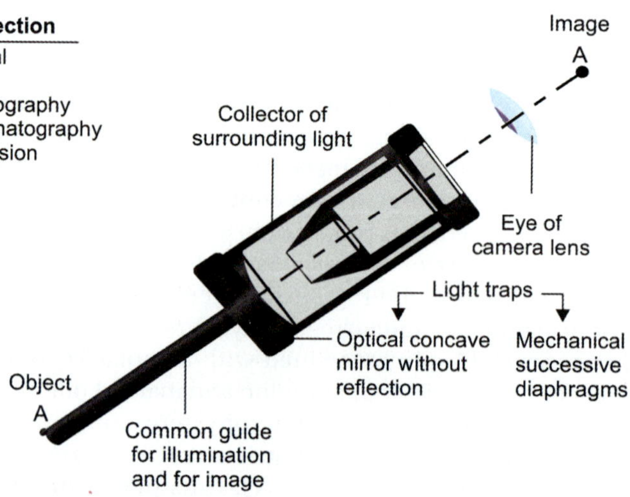

Fig. 3: The contact hysteroscope.

Source: The Institut d'Optique de Paris and manufactured by the MTO Company, Paris

the instrument must be maneuvered to give complete visualization of the endocervical canal and endometrial cavity. Tactile sensations are as important as the visual picture, because tissue may be distorted by undue pressure by the instrument.

Advantages and Disadvantages

Advantages are simplicity and independence from a connecting external light source. Also it may be used when there is bleeding, which does not interfere with visualization.

Disadvantage is the lack of a panoramic view of the endometrial cavity. Visual findings must therefore be interpreted as seen in 6 mm or 8 mm segments. Another disadvantage of the technique is that direct biopsy is impossible.

Applications

It can be used for diagnostic examinations similar to conventional hysteroscopy, including intrauterine device (IUD) localization, detection of uterine polyps and hyperplastic conditions of the endometrium, visualization of uterine synechiae, and identification of submucus fibroids.

In addition, to visualize the interior of the postpartum and the pregnant uterus and to check the completeness of a uterine curettage.

Also, to explore an intact pregnancy, the developing embryo can often be seen through the intact fetal membranes.

It can be used to examine vagina and cervix in infants and children.

Use of the instrument for the diagnosis and staging of adenocarcinoma of the endometrium holds promise, because a hysteroscopic diagnosis may be obtained without the potential danger of disseminating malignant cells to the peritoneal cavity through the tubes.

OFFICE HYSTEROSCOPY (FIG. 4)

To avoid anesthesia and hospital admission, to reduce the load on over stretched bed occupancy and precious operation theater time, and to reduce inconvenience of the patient wanting to get back to her daily routine quickly this procedure is now done as office procedure on outpatient basis using a conventional hysteroscope.

The introduction of small-caliber endoscopes [outer diameter (OD) less than 4 mm] that do not require cervical dilatation for their introduction in the uterus, facilitated the use of hysteroscopy in the office setting.[11,12] The small-caliber endoscope simplifies the examination and permits practical, safe, and efficient investigation of the uterine cavity.

The examination can be performed in a simpler, faster, and cleaner way, decreasing the need for anesthesia and/or analgesia. Nonetheless, it has inherent drawbacks. Owing to the relatively small diameter, no instrument can be passed through the small hysteroscope, as it is not usually fitted with

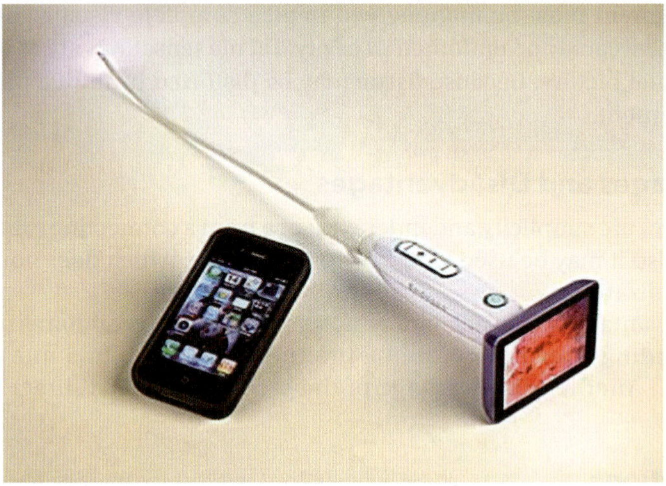

Fig. 4: Office hysteroscopy.

an operating channel. With these hysteroscopes, only CO_2 gas can be used as a practical medium to distend the uterine cavity adequately.

Newer endoscopes have a 4–5 mm OD, permitting continuous flow of a low-viscosity fluid via a small, built-in channel as well as the performance of minor operative procedures. These endoscopes can also be used in the office, permitting minor surgical procedures.

Routine use of opiate analgesia before outpatient hysteroscopy should be avoided as it may cause adverse effects. Routine cervical preparation before outpatient hysteroscopy should not be used.

The incidence of uterine trauma is low for diagnostic outpatient hysteroscopy performed with small-diameter endoscopes (outer sheath diameter under 5.5 mm) under direct vision.

Miniature hysteroscopes (2.7 mm with a 3–3.5 mm sheath) should be used for diagnostic outpatient hysteroscopy as they significantly reduce the discomfort experienced by the woman. There is insufficient evidence to recommend 0° or forward-oblique optical lenses (i.e. 12°, 25°, or 30° off-set lenses) for routine outpatient hysteroscopy. Choice of hysteroscope should be left to the discretion of the operator.

Flexible hysteroscopes are associated with less pain during outpatient hysteroscopy compared with rigid hysteroscopes. However, rigid hysteroscopes may provide better images, fewer failed procedures, quicker examination time, and reduced cost (Fig. 5).

Uterine distension with normal saline allows improved image quality and allows outpatient diagnostic hysteroscopy to be completed more quickly compared with carbon dioxide. The endoscope is introduced at the external os atraumatically and advanced until the uterine cavity is visualized. The advantage of this method is a continuous flow that washes away any debris, blood clots, or mucus that may impair visualization.[13] Operative outpatient

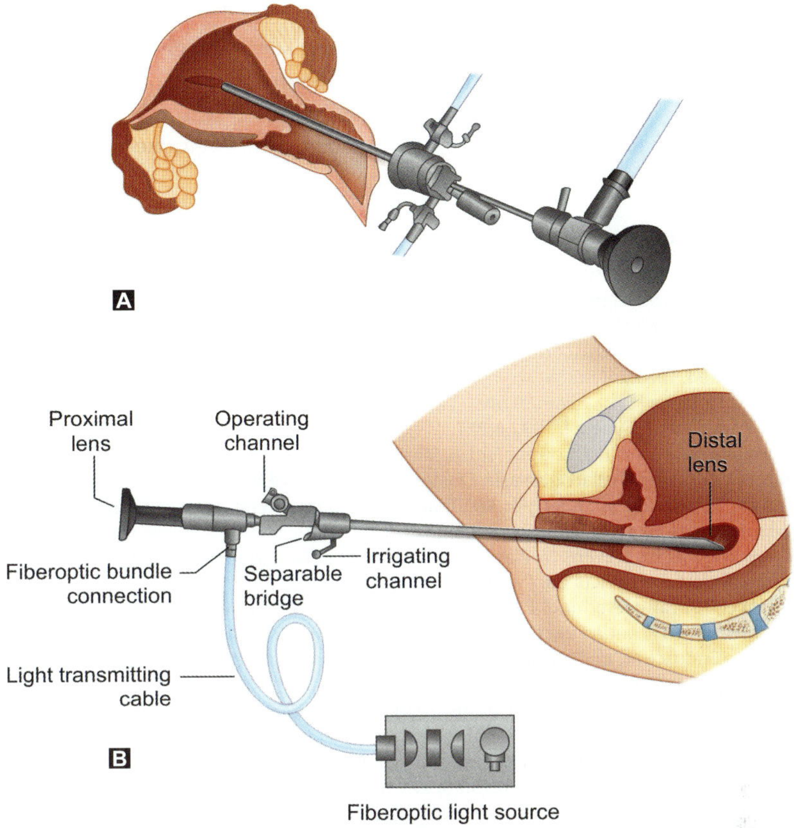

Figs. 5A and B: (A) Rigid hysteroscope, (B) Parts of rigid hysteroscope.

hysteroscopy, using bipolar electrosurgery, requires the use of normal saline to act as both the distension and conducting medium.

Routine cervical dilatation is associated with pain, vasovagal reactions and uterine trauma and should be avoided. Instillation of local anesthetic into the cervical canal does not reduce pain during diagnostic outpatient hysteroscopy but may reduce the incidence of vasovagal reactions.

Conscious sedation should not be routinely used in outpatient hysteroscopic procedures as it confers no advantage in terms of pain control and the woman's satisfaction over local anesthesia.

It offers:

- A familiar and comfortable environment for the procedure
- Saved time for patient and physician
- Saved money for the patient with a large deductible or coinsurance
- No requirement for general anesthesia
- Local anesthesia can be used, but is not necessary
- Immediate visual affirmation for the patient and physician
- A see and treat possibility

- Possibility of preoperative decision-making
- Use in menopausal and nulliparous patients with no cervical preparation necessary when a small-diameter hysteroscope or flexible hysteroscope is used
- Minimized discomfort from a speculum with the vaginoscopic approach for awake patients.

REFERENCES

1. Hamou JE. Microhysteroscopie: Une nouvelle technique en endoscopie, ses applications. Acta Endoscopica. 1980;10(5-6):415-22.
2. Hamou JE. Microhysteroscopy: A new procedure and its original applications in gynecology. J Reprod Med. 1981;26(7):376-82.
3. Hamou JE, Taylor PJ. Panoramic contact and microcolpohysteroscopy in gynecologic practice. Curr Probl Obstet Gynecol. 1982;6(2):1.
4. Hamou JE, Sala-Baroux J, Coupez F, et al. Microhysteroscopy: A new approach to the diagnosis of cervical intraepithelial neoplasia. Obstet Gynecol. 1984;63(4):567-74.
5. Hamou JE, Sala-Baroux J, Siegler AM. Diagnosis and treatment of intrauterine adhesions by microhysteroscopy. Fertil Steril. 1983;39(3):321-6.
6. Van Herendael BJ, Stevens M, Flakiewicz-Kuler A, et al. Dating of the endometrium by micro-colpo-hysteroscopy. Acta Eur Fertil. 1986;17:451.
7. Bettocchi S, Van Herendael BJ, Colafranceschi M, et al. Un nuovo quadro inisteroscopia diagnostica: 1o Pseudo Functional Dysvascular Endometrium. G Ital Ost Gin. 1993;15:592.
8. David C. Endoscopic de l'uterus apres l'avortement et dans les suites de couches normales et pathologiques. Bull Soc Obstet Paris. 1907;10:288.
9. Parent B, Tougas C, Doerler B. L'hysteroscopie de contact. J Gynecol Obstet Biol Reprod. 1974;3:511.
10. Barbot J. Contact hysteroscopy: Another method of endoscopic examination of the uterine cavity. Am J Obstet Gynecol. 1980;136(6):721-6
11. Font-Sastre V, Carabias J, Bonilla-Musoles F, et al. Office hysteroscopy with small calibre instruments: Proceedings of the Second World Congress on Hysteroscopy. Acta Eur Fertil. 1986;17:427.
12. Valle RF. Future of office hysteroscopy. In Isaacson KB (Ed): Office Hysteroscopy. St Louis: Mosby Year Book; 1996. pp. 117-30.
13. Valle RF. Office hysteroscopy. Clin Obstet Gynecol. 1999;42(2):276-89.

Chapter 5

Hysteroscopic Evaluation of Infertile Couple

PC Mahapatra

INTRODUCTION

Infertility is a life crisis. The number of couples seeking medical help for infertility is increasing dramatically. The incidence of infertility in any community varies between 5% and 15%.

It is widely accepted that a complete infertility workup should include an evaluation of the uterine cavity. Uterine abnormalities, congenital or acquired, are implicated as one of the causes of infertility. In fact, infertility related to uterine cavity abnormalities has been estimated to be the causal factor in as many as 10–15% of couples seeking treatment. Moreover, abnormal uterine findings have been found in 34–62% of infertile women.[1]

One of the basic steps of an infertility workup is to evaluate the shape and regularity of the uterine cavity. Acquired uterine lesions, such as uterine fibroids, endometrial polyps, intrauterine adhesions, or all of these, may cause infertility by interfering with proper embryo implantation and growth.[1]

Congenital uterine malformations are also thought to play a role in delaying natural conception.[1]

SCOPE OF THE HYSTEROSCOPY

Many authors believe that uterine and endometrial integrity should be evaluated primarily by hysteroscopy in the infertile or in vitro fertilization (IVF)-treated population.[15]

During the last two decades several studies have demonstrated that when the uterine cavity has to be investigated within the infertility workup, hysteroscopy is much more accurate than hysterosalpingography (HSG).[2,4,5,8] Kessler and Lancet reported that in about two-thirds of the cases hysteroscopy findings were not correlated with those found on HSG.[4-7]

INDICATIONS OF HYSTEROSCOPY IN INFERTILITY MANAGEMENT

The most common indication is as a part of initial infertility workup. Other indications are as a part of continuous infertility workup, before IVF treatment and after a number of failed IVF cycles.[8,14]

It helps in detecting possible intrauterine changes that could interfere with implantation or growth, or both, of the conceptus, and in evaluating the benefit of different treatment modalities in restoring a normal endometrial environment[(c)].

Different hypotheses have been suggested to define the mechanism of infertility due to intrauterine pathologies. Polyps may cause infertility by virtue of their location, thereby causing mechanical block (e.g. tubocornual polyp) by their association with endometriosis, or by expression of the enzyme aromatase. Myomas that protrude into the cavity may decrease vascular supply to the trophoblastic tissue when implantation takes place on the overlying endometrium. Most septa are relatively avascular and hence result in implantation failure when implantation takes place over them. Other pathologies like synechiae, endometritis, cervical stenosis, and chronic cervicitis can be causes of subfertility (Figs. 1A to D).

ABNORMALITIES OF THE UTERINE CAVITY

The abnormalities of the endometrial cavity can be congenital or acquired.

Congenital Anomalies

These anomalies occur in 3–4% of all women. This increases to 5–10% in women with early pregnancy losses and up to 25% in those with second and third trimester losses. The incidence of uterine malformations in other series of infertile patients varies between 1% and 26%, with a mean incidence of 3.4%.[3]

While the relationship between congenital uterine malformations and impaired pregnancy outcome (such as recurrent pregnancy loss, late abortions, preterm deliveries, and malpresentations) is quite established, the issue of these malformations as a cause of infertility is still debatable.

Septate or bicornuate uterus is the most common anomaly found.

In spite of the comprehensive study of infertility, little data are available concerning the benefit of different treatment protocols after septum resection on fertility consequence. Most of the researchers have shown a better reproductive outcome after hysteroscopic resection of uterine septum in woman with septate uterus; however, there is no evidence on the postoperative management of the hysteroscopic septum division.

Nouri et al. represented an overall pregnancy rate of 60.1% and a live-birth rate of 45% after hysteroscopic metroplasty.[16] Studies by Pabuccu R et al. (2004), Shokeir et al. (2011), and Paradisi R et al. (2013) show similar findings.[17,18]

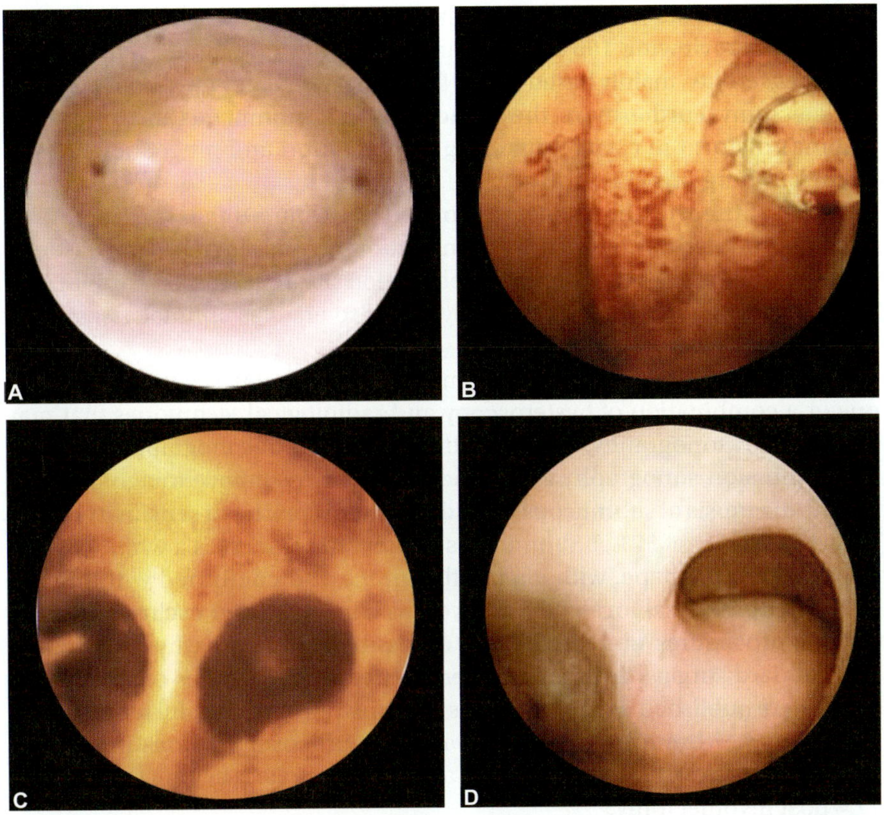

Figs. 1A to D: (A) A normal uterus; (B) A uterus with a large polyp; (C) Uterus divided by septum; (D) Uterus with a fibroid.

In a retrospective, matched, controlled study, the role of septate uterus in the reproductive performance of patients requiring IVF was evaluated. The pregnancy rate before metroplasty was lower than after metroplasty, and the abortion rate was higher. They suggest that the presence of septate uterus, may be, decreased the pregnancy rate and increased the abortion rate after the embryo transfers for IVF/intracytoplasmic sperm injection.[19]

Acquired Abnormalities of the Uterus

Leiomyomas

These benign monoclonal uterine myometrial tumors affect 25–45% of reproductive age women. The mechanisms by which uterine fibroids cause infertility are unknown but may involve altered uterine contractility, impaired gamete transport, or endometrial dysfunction. Subserosal fibroids do not appear to affect fertility or obstetric outcomes whereas, intramural and submucosal myomas appear to lower implantation and live birth rates.

Donnez and Jadoul tried to address the issue "whether myomas influence fertility", by reviewing 106 relevant articles.[21] They concluded that they do influence fertility, mainly based on the favorable pregnancy rates obtained after myomectomy. Furthermore, they concluded that submucous and intramural myomas distort the cavity, impairing implantation and pregnancy rates in women undergoing IVF.

Several theories have been proposed regarding this issue, including alteration of uterine contractility or induction of inflammatory and vascular changes leading to a less receptive implantation site. Hysteroscopy cannot only diagnose these pathologies accurately, but also enables optimal assessment for possible myomectomy.[22]

The diagnosis of submucous leiomyomas is generally accomplished with one or a combination of hysteroscopy and radiological techniques that may include ultrasonography, [typically transvaginal ultrasonography (TVUS)], saline infusion sonography (SIS), and magnetic resonance imaging (MRI). For the diagnosis of submucous fibroids, hysteroscopy has a sensitivity of 82% and a specificity of 87%.[20] Submucous leiomyoma is seen as a white-colored bulge, round in shape, with a smooth surface and confirmed with biopsy. In their submucosal localization, myomas can be treated exclusively using surgical procedures, and they may be accessible by operative hysteroscopy—the standard surgical approach. Several retrospective studies of small cases series were published during the 1990s demonstrating successful reproductive outcome after hysteroscopic removal of submucosal myomas in infertile women. Authors have reported clinical pregnancy rates ranging from 31% to 77% post myomectomy.

Fluid overload and uterine perforation are the most common complications of hysteroscopic myomectomy (Table 1).

Endometrial Polyp

The incidence of asymptomatic endometrial polyps in women with infertility has been reported to range from 6% to 8%, but may be as high as 32%. Nevertheless, Shokeir found such lesions to be more frequent in the unexplained infertility population compared with fertile women.

The impact of polyps on infertility is mainly dependent on their size and location. A prospective randomized study of the impact of polyps on an IVF program, by Lass et al.,[23] concluded that small endometrial polyp (less than 2 cm) do not decrease the pregnancy rate after IVF, but a trend toward increased pregnancy loss exists.

Hysteroscopy with guided biopsy is the most common comparator for other techniques to diagnose polyps as it offers the highest sensitivity and specificity for conservative measures. Diagnostic hysteroscopy alone only allows subjective assessment of the size and characteristic of the lesion with reported sensitivity of 58–99%, specificity of 87–100%, PPV of 21–100, and NPV of 66–99% when compared with hysteroscopy with guided biopsy.[25] These

Table 1: Summary of studies reporting on the reproductive outcome after hysteroscopic myomectomy.

Author	*No. of cases*	*No. of pregnancies*	*Pregnancy rate (%)*	*Delivery rate (%)*
Donnez *et al* (1990)	24	16	67	67
Valle (1990)	16	10	62	50
Corson and Brooks (1991)	13	10	77	61
Hucke (1992)	14	4	28.7	–
Goldenberg *et al* (1995)	15	7	47	40
Preutthipan and Theppisai (1998)	12	2	16.7	–
Giatras *et al* (1999)	41	25	60.9	48.7
Varasteh *et al* (1999)	36	19	52.8	36.1

appear as small growths in the uterine cavity which are soft, oval, pedunculated with a smooth surface.

Menstrual pattern was normalized in the majority of patients after hysteroscopic polypectomy. In addition, hysteroscopic polypectomy is a safe procedure with low complication rate.[24] Removal of these polyps may enhance reproductive outcome.

Intrauterine Synechiae or Asherman's Syndrome

Severe trauma to the basalis layer of the endometrium with subsequent tissue bridge formation leads to synechiae or Asherman's syndrome. The causes of intrauterine adhesions are often iatrogenic with patients typically reporting intraoperative or postoperative complications following uterine evacuations for incomplete pregnancy loss or postpartum hemorrhage or pregnancy termination. In developing countries like India, Asherman's syndrome due to genital tuberculosis is quite common.

This is one of the most common causes of secondary infertility. In spite of the known relationship between secondary infertility and the existence of adhesions, no significant difference was found in the rate of intrauterine adhesions comparing the patients with primary versus secondary infertility. Oliveira[9] also found intrauterine adhesions in 10% of patients with repeated filed IVF cycles of whom none had undergone previous abortions or other uterine manipulation. Hysteroscopy is the gold standard for diagnosis and treatment of intrauterine adhesions. A combination of blunt and sharp dissection or electrosurgery is used by most units. Treatment should follow a protocol that incorporates sound hysteroscopic technique with antibiotic prophylaxis and postoperative hormonal therapy. Consideration should be given to the use of an intrauterine contraceptive device or Foley catheter for a short period.

The NICE guideline on fertility treatment published in 2004 recommends that "Women with amenorrhea who are found to have intrauterine adhesions should be offered hysteroscopic adhesiolysis because this is likely to restore menstruation and improve the chance of pregnancy".

Though transvaginal ultrasound, HSG and hysteroscopy are complementary in the evaluation of the infertile patient. Hysteroscopy can diagnose small intrauterine lesions much more precisely (compared with HSG and even TVS) and treat them simultaneously. Based on the results of the previous studies, it appears that more than one-third of the patients interpreted as normal following HSG are found to have a uterine abnormality after diagnostic hysteroscopy, which might be a significant cause of reproductive failure. These women may be wrongly treated, or unnecessarily investigated, while their intrauterine lesion has been missed.

Furthermore, hysteroscopy allows exact location of intrauterine lesions, and provides a better way than the blunt curettage to ensure excision of such lesions.[11,12]

HYSTEROSCOPY IN ARTIFICIAL REPRODUCTIVE TECHNIQUE

Despite advances in the field of artificial reproductive techniques over the past 20 years, implantation rates per embryo transferred still remain low, at about 15–20%.[13] The two key factors in question for this problem are the quality of the embryo and the receptivity of the uterus.

Although it is possible to assess the embryo quality by microscopy, uterine receptivity cannot be fully evaluated.

Currently, the *European Society of Human Reproduction and Embryology (ESHRE)* guidelines indicate hysteroscopy to be unnecessary, unless it is for the confirmation and treatment of doubtful intrauterine pathology.[10] Nevertheless, in a study by Shoker et al. it was suggested that 26% of the patients with normal HSG were with abnormal hysteroscopic findings.[13] The role of hysteroscopy in patients undergoing IVF seems to be vital for patients in whom an IVF is being contemplated, for treatment of infertility. Intrauterine pathologies and structural uterine abnormalities that may be responsible for the failure of IVF can be detected and treated, resulting in improved pregnancy rates.

Oliveira reported detection of significant, unsuspected intrauterine abnormalities, found only with hysteroscopy, in 25% of patients with repeated failed in vitro fertilization and embryo transfer (IVF-ET) cycles.[9] All of his patient population had normal HSG within the former year. More importantly, relevant therapeutic interventions significantly improved the clinical pregnancy rate in those with abnormal uterine cavity at hysteroscopy.

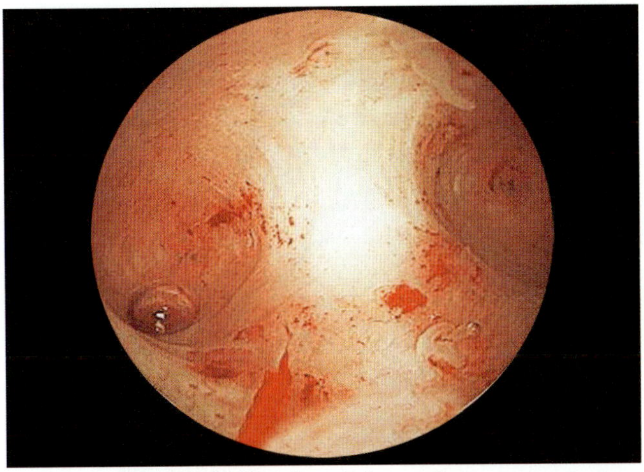

Fig. 2: Showing uterine septum.

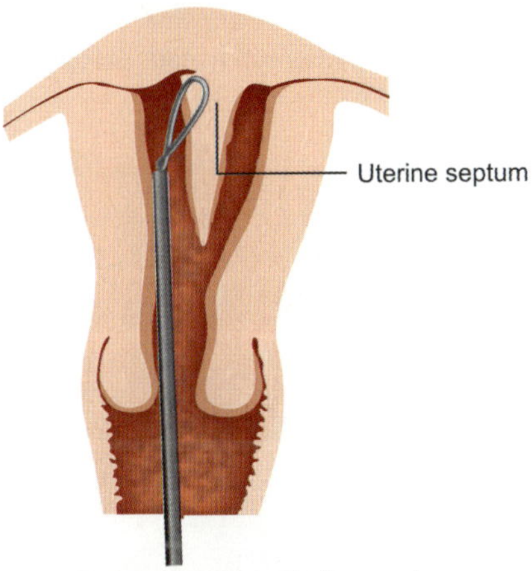

Fig. 3: Showing uterine septum.

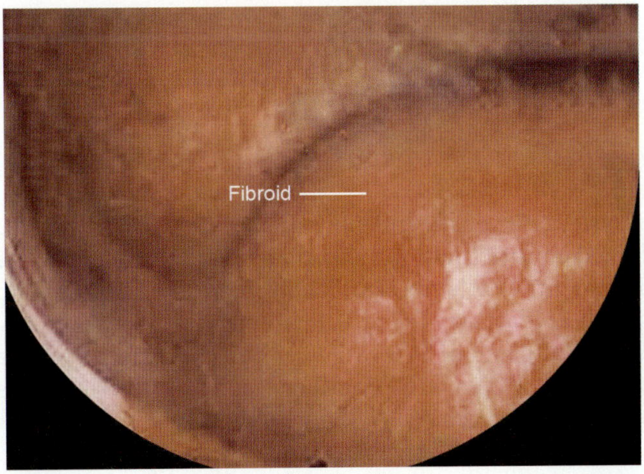

Fig. 4: Showing fibroid.

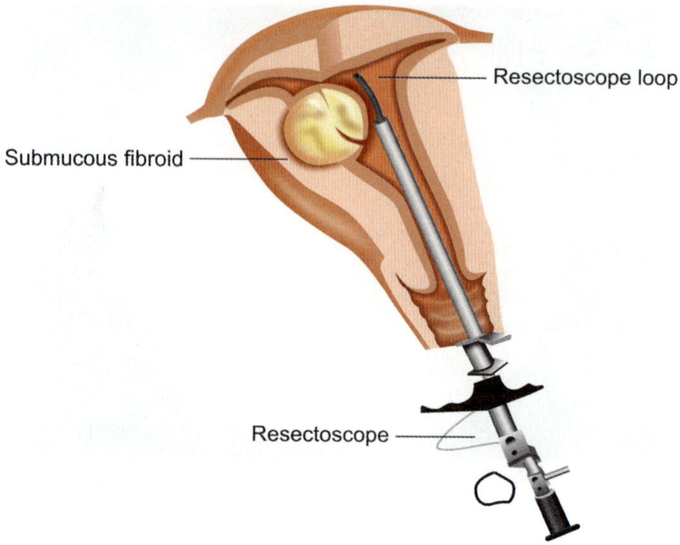

Fig. 5: Showing submucous fibroid.

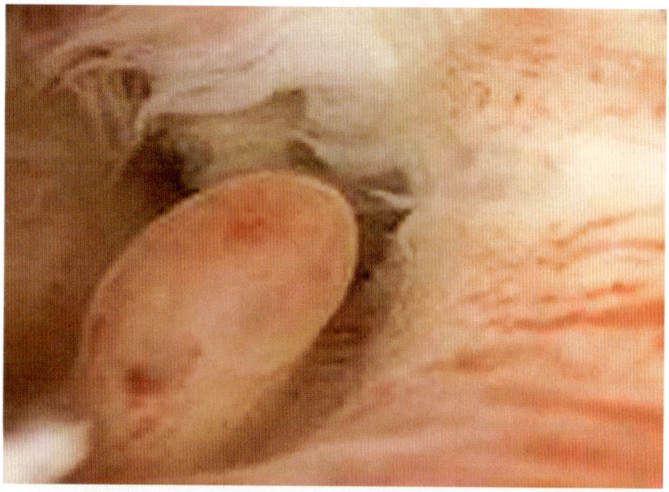

Fig. 6: Endometrial polyp.

The role of hysteroscopy in patients with previously failed IVF cycles has been studied.

A recent systematic review and meta-analysis of two randomized and three nonrandomized control trials on 1,691 patients concluded that hysteroscopy before a subsequent IVF attempt significantly increases the odds for conception in patients with at least two failed IVF attempts.[10] This would also save the patient additional costs of IVF cycles, where failures occur because the intrauterine pathology is missed on other screening investigations like HSG. This is especially true in women with one or more prior failed IVF cycles.

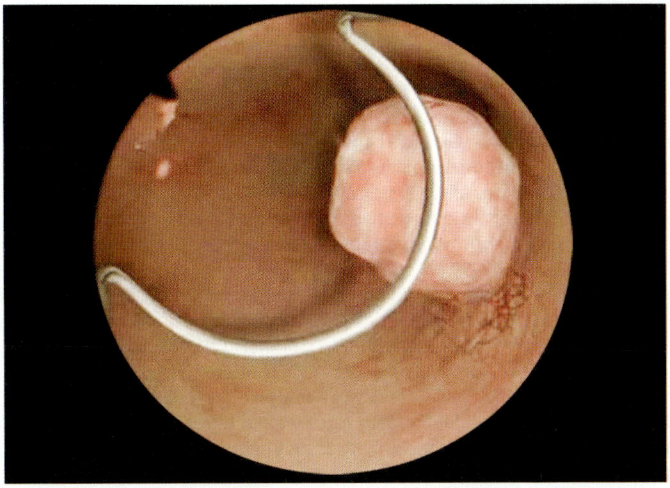

Fig. 7: Resectoscope with fibroid.

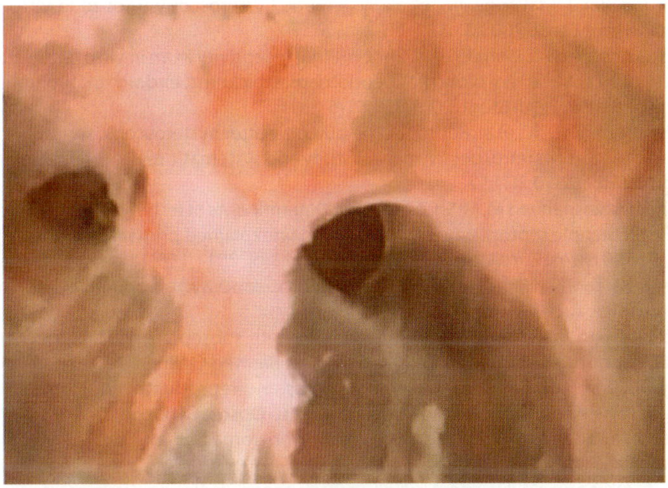

Fig. 8: Showing septum.

Thus routine hysteroscopy should be included in the evaluation of the infertile couple.

REFERENCES

1. Brown SE, Coddington CC, Schnorr J, et al. Evaluation of outpatient hysteroscopy, saline infusion hysterosonography and hysterosalpingography in infertile women: a prospective, randomized study. Fertil Steril. 2000;74:1029-34.
2. Prevedourakis C, Loutradis D, Kalianidis C, et al. Hysterosalpingography and hysteroscopy in female infertility. Hum Reprod. 1994;9(12):2353-5.

3. Pansky M, Feingold M, Sagi R, et al. Diagnostic hysteroscopy as a primary tool in a basic infertility workup. JSLS. 2006;10(2):231-5.
4. Golan A, Eilat E, Ron-El R, et al. Hysteroscopy is superior to hysterosalpingography in infertility investigation. Acta Obstet Gynecol Scand. 1996;75:654-6.
5. Wang CW, Lee CL, Lai YM, et al. Comparison of hysterosalpingography and hysteroscopy in female infertility. J Am Assoc Gynecol Laparosc. 1996;3:581-4.
6. Brooks PG, Serden SP. Hysteroscopic findings after unsuccessful dilatation and curettage for abnormal uterine bleeding. Am J Obstet Gynecol. 1988;158:1354-7.
7. Kung F, Chen W, Chou H, et al. Conservative management of early endometrial adenocarcinoma with repeat curettage and hormone therapy under assistance of hysteroscopy and laparoscopy. Hum Reprod. 1997;12:1649-53.
8. Kessler I, Lancet M. Hysterography and hysteroscopy: a comparison. Fertil Steril. 1986;46:709-10.
9. Grimbizis GF, Camus M, Tarlatzis BS, et al. Clinical implications of uterine malformations and hysteroscopic treatment results. Hum Reprod Update. 2001;7(1):161-74.
10. El Toukhy T, Sunkara SK, Coomarasamy A, et al. Outpatient hysteroscopy and subsequent IVF cycle outcome: A systematic review and meta-analysis. Reprod Biomed Online. 2008;16:712-9.
11. Salle B, Bied Damon V, et al. Preliminary report of an ultrasonography and colour Doppler uterine score to predict uterine receptivity in an in vitro fertilization program. Hum Reprod. 1998;13:1669-73.
12. Crosignani PG, Rubin BL. Optimal use of infertility diagnostic tests and treatments: The ESHRE Capri Workshop Group. Hum Reprod. 2000;15:723-32.
13. Shokeir TA, Shalan HM, El Shafei MN. Significance of endometrial polyps detected hysteroscopically in infertile women. J Obstet Gynecol. 2004;30:84-9.
14. Faghali J, Bakar J, Mayenga JM, et al. Systematic hysteroscopy prior to in vitro fertilisation. Gynecol Obstet Fertil. 2003;31:127-31.
15. Schild RL, Knobloch C, Dorn C, et al. Endometrial receptivity in an in vitro fertilisation program as assessed by spiral artery blood flow, endometrial thickness, endometrial volume and uterine artery blood flow. Fertil Steril. 2001;75:361-6.
16. Nouri K, Ott J, Huber JC, et al. Reproductive outcome after hysteroscopic septoplasty in patients with septate uterus-a retrospective cohort study and systematic review of the literature. Reprod Biol Endocrinol. 2010;8(1):52.
17. Shokeir T, Abdelshaheed M, El-Shafie M, et al. Determinants of fertility and reproductive success after hysteroscopic septoplasty for women with unexplained primary infertility: a prospective analysis of 88 cases. Eur J Obstet Gynecol Reprod Biol. 2011;155(1):54-7.
18. Paradisi R, Barzanti R, Natali F, et al. Hysteroscopic metroplasty: reproductive outcome in relation to septum size. Arch Gynecol Obstet. 2013:1-6.
19. Tomaževič T, Ban-Frangež H, Virant-Klun I, et al. Septate, subseptate and arcuate uterus decrease pregnancy and live birth rates in IVF/ICSI. Reprod Biomed Online. 2010;21(5):700-5.
20. Klatsky PC, Tran ND, Caughey AB, et al. Fibroids and reproductive outcomes: a systematic literature review from conception to delivery. Am J Obstet Gynecol. 2008;198:357-66.
21. Donnez J, Jadoul P. What are the implications of myomas on infertility? A need for debate? Hum Reprod. 2002;17(6):1424-30.
22. Nagele F, O'Connor H, Davies A, et al. 2500 outpatient diagnostic hysteroscopies. Obstet Gynecol. 1996;88:87-92.
23. Lass A, Williams G, Abusheikha N, et al. The effect of endometrial polyps on outcomes of in vitro fertilization (IVF) cycles. J Assist Reprod Genet. 1999;16(8):410-5.
24. Stamatellos I, Apostolides A, Stamatopoulos P, et al. Pregnancy rates after hysteroscopic polypectomy depending on the size or number of the polyps. Arch Gynecol Obstet. 2008;277(5):395-9.
25. American Association of Gynecologic Laparoscopists. AAGL practice report: practice guidelines for the diagnosis and management of endometrial polyp. J Minim Invasive Gynecol. 2012;19(1):3-10.

Chapter 6

Hysteroscopy in Abnormal Uterine Bleeding

Nahata VS, Bhardwaj F, Mittal M

INTRODUCTION

Abnormal uterine bleeding (AUB) is a common problem among women in the reproductive age. AUB may be accompanied by pain and discomfort, has a substantial effect on health-related quality of life, and causes significant social embarrassment. AUB leads to loss of productivity and may result in surgical interventions including hysterectomy. Management of such common condition in a population with wide healthcare diversity requires uniform clinical practice guidelines.

Diagnosis of AUB requires meticulous history taking, thorough clinical examination, necessary investigations and imaging. For years, ultrasound (US) has been the standard imaging technique in case of AUB. Plenty of diagnostic techniques [such as transvaginal ultrasound (TVS), TVS with saline solution infusion, dilation and curettage (D&C), and endometrial biopsy] have been widely used in order to evaluate women with AUB. Hysteroscopy has opened up new diagnostic vistas for the diagnostic evaluation of the cervical canal and uterine cavity, revealing the inherent limits of dilation, curettage, and endometrial biopsy if performed without visual guidance. Moreover, hysteroscopy has emerged as an important tool for diagnosis and treatment for endocervical and intracavitary lesions of uterus.

To develop consistency and universally acceptable nomenclature of AUB, FIGO (International Federation of Gynecology and Obstetrics) has given PALM-COEIN (polyp, adenomyosis, leiomyoma, malignancy, and hyperplasia-coagulopathy, ovulatory dysfunction, endometrial, iatrogenic, and not yet classified) classification (Fig. 1).

The advent of recent technical innovations has revolutionized the field of hysteroscopy, making it possible to perform a comprehensive endoscopic examination of the uterine cavity in an outpatient session, without using any type of anesthetic or preliminary dilatation of the cervical canal. As a consequence, the indication range for hysteroscopic procedures has been extended considerably. The hysteroscopic technique is indicated in all

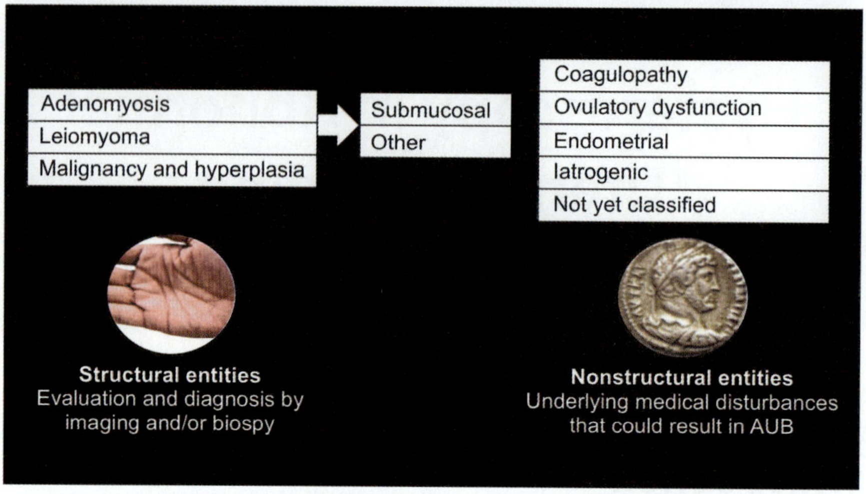

Fig. 1: PALM-COEIN classification given by FIGO for AUB.
(**PALM-COEIN:** Polyp, adenomyosis, leiomyoma, malignancy, and hyperplasia-coagulopathy, ovulatory dysfunction, endometrial, iatrogenic, and not yet classified; FIGO: International Federation of Gynecology and Obstetrics; AUB: abnormal uterine bleeding).

those cases that require direct visualization of the cervical canal and uterine cavity. Diagnostic and surgical hysteroscopy have become gold standards in gynecological practice.

Plenty of authors till today have managed to demonstrate the great potential of hysteroscopy as the gold standard method for the investigation of women with such pathology. Barati et al. have announced that in a sum of 147 women with AUB and normal TVS, 32 of them (21.8%) were hysteroscopically abnormal and cervical canal polyp has been described as the commonest lesion that has been misdiagnosed by TVS. Endometrial or cervical polyps can be treated better by hysteroscopy since D&C has proved to be less effective. A few years earlier, Refaie et al. evaluated 112 pre- and postmenopausal women with AUB in order to assess if an outpatient hysteroscopy affects the decision making of treatment. The authors concluded that half of the women had abnormal uterine cavities with most common findings of the submucous myomas and endometrial polyps, and that hysteroscopical investigation of AUB could lead to the most appropriate treatment, without unnecessary major surgical intervention. Bettocchi et al. have proved the efficacy of office hysteroscopy treatment in benign intrauterine pathologies in menopausal women. He has enrolled in his study a sum of 925 menopausal women with AUB in a period of 5 years and divided them into two investigation groups according to the endometrial thickness (group 1 <4 mm and group 2 >4 mm). The conclusion was that the diagnostic value of hysteroscopy yielded 99–100% specificity and sensitivity respectively for both groups.

The most frequent hysteroscopic findings in patients with AUB are the submucous myomas, polyps, and endometrial hyperplasia, either benign or malignant, in about 60–70% of the cases.

The most common type of pelvic malignancy still remains the endometrial cancer. This type of malignancy causes abnormal genital bleeding usually as a first symptom in most of the cases, thus, the early investigation of such symptom is of great importance for a woman's survival and progress. Unfortunately, some of the women with endometrial adenocarcinoma remain asymptomatic. Endometrial hyperplasia is deemed as a precursor of endometrial cancer. The most important sign of endometrial cancer or endometrial hyperplasia is the endometrial thickness in an US exam. Unfortunately, US exam has very low specificity in the differentiation of the type of endometrial hyperplasia as soon as directed biopsy of the suspected uterus still remains a prerequisite for an appropriate control. An endometrial thickness greater than 4 mm requires further evaluation in postmenopausal women with AUB. Hysteroscopy not only can clearly and accurately display the appearance of endometrial cancer but also demonstrates any possible involvement of the lower uterine segment and cervix. Endometrial hyperplasia is an overgrowth of endometrial glands, with different shapes and sizes, which causes increased endometrial thickness which results in a greater gland/stroma ratio (>50%) than observed in normal endometrium.

CLASSIFICATION

World Health Organization (WHO) Classification

The 2015 WHO endometrial hyperplasia classification system has only two categories:

1. Hyperplasia without atypia (nonneoplastic)
2. Atypical hyperplasia (endometrial intraepithelial neoplasm).

Hysteroscopic finding of endometrial hyperplasia is:

- Hyperplasia without atypia (Fig. 2)
  - Increased endometrial thickness (resembling normal one)
  - Presence of cystic dilatation
  - Polyploid formation (complex one)
  - Increased vascularization (rich but regular vessels).
- Hyperplasia with atypia (Fig. 3)
  - Irregular and polyploidal growth with abnormal vascularization (Arborizing vessels or corkscrew vessels). It can be described as "cereb irregular brain surface"
  - Endometrium bleeds very easily on touch
  - Unfortunately, it is difficult to differentiate between complex endometrial hyperplasia and endometrial adenocarcinoma
  - There is no consensus on the hysteroscopic appearance of endometrial hyperplasia.

There are four hysteroscopic patterns of endometrial adenocarcinoma:

1. Polypoid
   - Histologically well-differentiated growth
   - Abnormal polyploidal endometrial growth

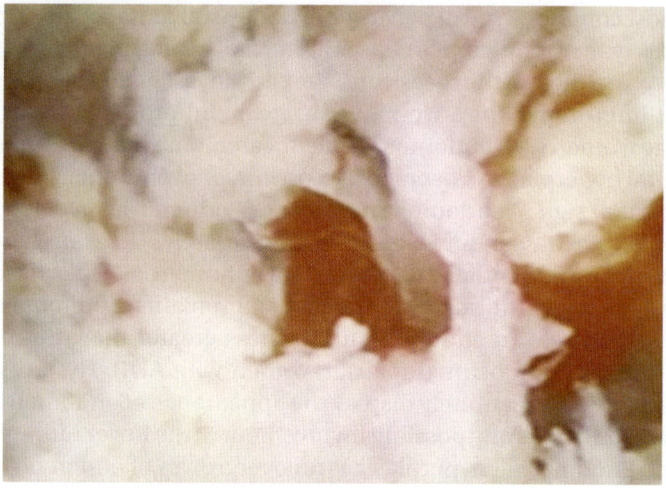

Fig. 2: Hyperplasia without atypia.

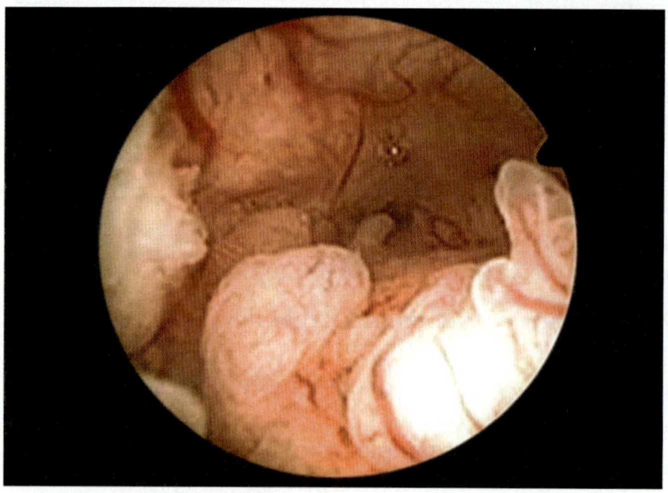

Fig. 3: Hyperplasia with atypia.

   - Abnormal vascularization (superficial arborescent vessels or corkscrew pattern).
2. Nodular (Figs. 4A and B)
   - Solid appearance
   - Marked atypical vascularization (Atypical vessels in zigzag form on the surface of the tumor).
3. Papillomatosis (Fig. 5)
   - Nodular appearance with the surface covered with numerous tentacle-like projection
   - Each projection is composed of a blood vessel covered with cancerous tissue.

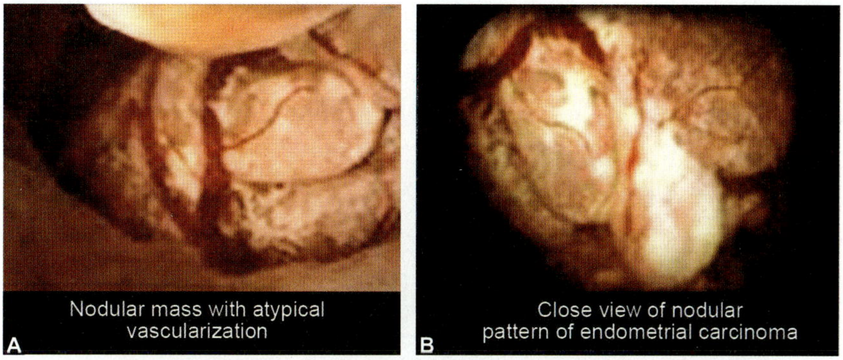

Figs. 4A and B: Nodular hysteroscopic pattern of endometrial adenocarcinoma.

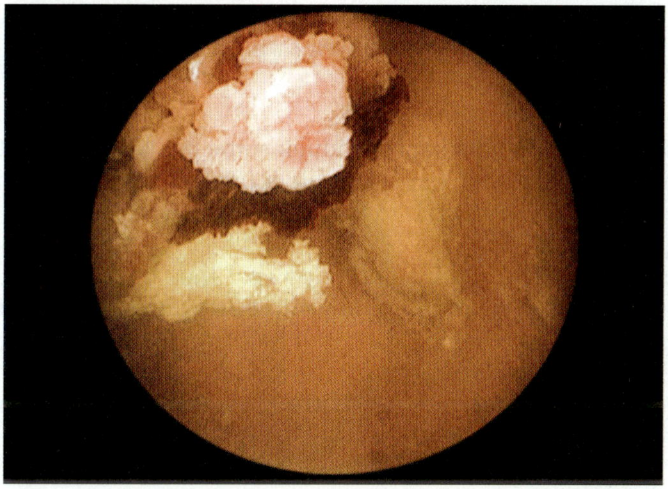

Fig. 5: Papillomatosis.

4. Diffuse carcinoma
   - Entire cavity is affected
   - Usually poorly differentiated.

Cordeiro and her colleagues summarized hysteroscopic findings in 245 postmenopausal women with increased endometrial thickness in TVS and compared the diagnostic outcomes regarding the presence or absence of AUB. In this study, the investigators suggested that sensitivity, specificity, positive predictive, and negative predictive value of hysteroscopy for endometrial carcinoma was 94.1%, 98.95%, 88.9%, and 99.5%, respectively.

ENDOMETRIAL POLYP

Overgrowth of cells in the lining of the uterus (endometrium) leads to the formation of uterine polyps, also known as endometrial polyps. These

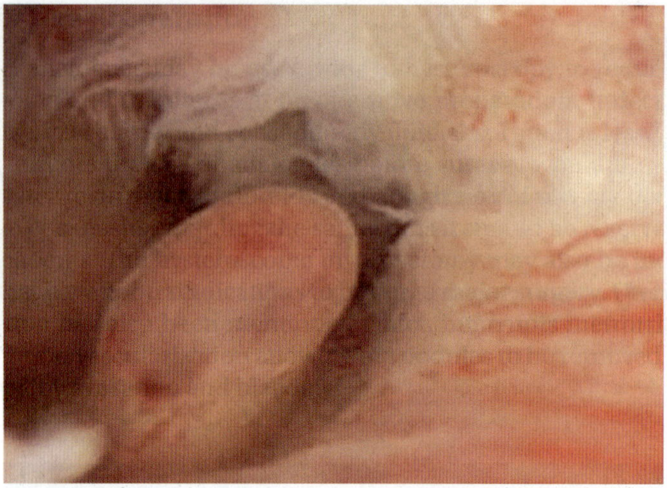

Fig. 6: Endometrial polyp.

polyps are usually premalignant, although some can be malignant. Uterine polyps range in size from a few millimeters (no larger than a sesame seed) to few centimeters. They attach to the uterine wall by a large base or a thin stalk (Fig. 6).

You can have one or many uterine polyps. They usually stay contained within uterus, but occasionally, they slip down through the opening of the uterus (cervix) into vagina. On hysteroscopy it looks like "tongue-like projection" into the uterine cavity.

It is common in women greater than 40 years and is a common cause of postmenopausal women.

SUBMUCOUS MYOMA

It can cause AUB, infertility, or recurrent pregnancy loss. Hysteroscopy is the gold standard in both diagnosis and treatment. On hysteroscopy, it looks like a round mass lesion with vessels seen upon the surface (Fig. 7).

Various classifications of submucous myoma are given by European Society for Gynaecological Endoscopy (ESGE).

ESGE Classification of Submucous Myomas (Fig. 8)

- Type 0
  - Entirely within endometrial cavity
  - No myometrial extension (pedunculated).
- Type I
  - Less than 50% myometrial extension (sessile)
  - Greater than 90 degree angle of myoma surface to uterine wall.

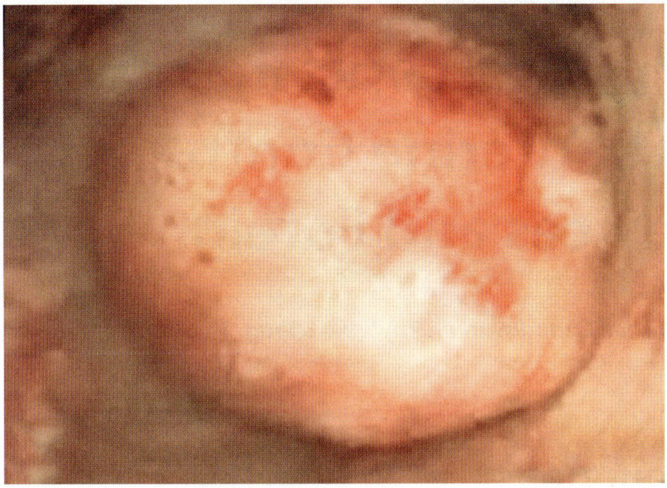

Fig. 7: Submucous myoma.

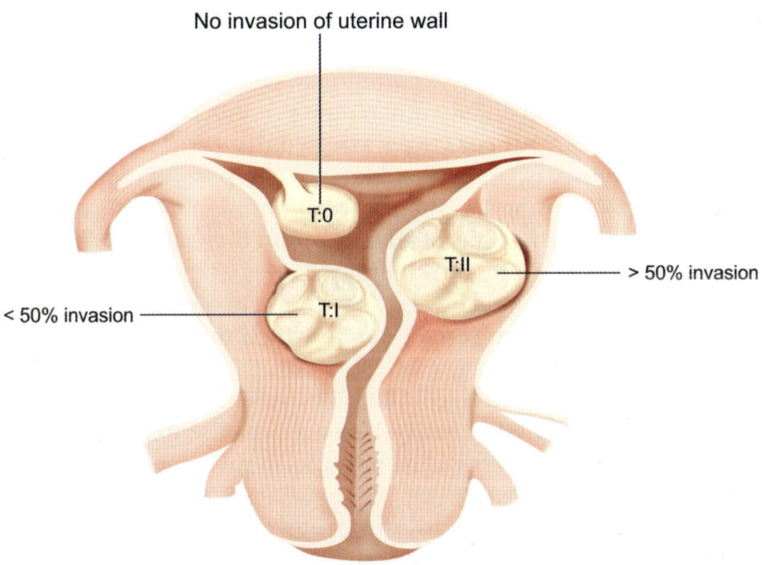

Fig. 8: European Society for Gynaecological Endoscopy (ESGE) classification of submucous myomas.

- Type II
  - Greater than or equal to 50% myometrial extension (sessile)
  - Greater than or equal to 90 degree angle of myoma surface to uterine wall.

Chapter 7

Hysteroscopic Removal of Intrauterine Contraceptive Devices and Foreign Bodies

Abhishek Chandavarkar, Priyanka Suhag, Madhura Chandavarkar

INTRODUCTION

A variety of foreign bodies have been described in literature in the genitourinary tract, from young girls to geriatric population. In the past, dealing with them was tedious task. Common foreign bodies encountered include tampon, pins, seeds, forgotten pessaries with presentation being vaginal discharge to infertility.[1,2] Foreign bodies are less common in uterine cavity than vagina and are less frequently seen in older women than prepubertal and premenarchal girls.[3] When found in uterus, they are usually forgotten intrauterine contraceptive device (IUCD), retained fetal bones, parts of conceptus, gauze pieces or parts of instruments. The most commonly found foreign body in uterus is lost IUCDs.[4-7] There has been case report on neglected fetal bones in the uterus for eight years after termination of pregnancy.[8]

As gynecologists, we would have at some point in our careers, come across a missing IUCD or a broken thread due to which the IUCD remains in the uterine cavity.

Most gynecologists would be comfortable in using a long artery forcep and blindly fishing out the missing IUCD. However, in case that blind procedure does not turn out to be successful, the next tool in the armamentarium would have to be the hysteroscope.

Prior to the era of hysteroscopy, this protocol may have been correct. In today's era, with hysteroscopy being available, patients need not undergo the painful blind access with an artery forcep. To make it even more feasible, office hysteroscopy can make it an outpatient department (OPD) procedure rather than even a day care procedure.

EQUIPMENT REQUIRED

- Endoscopy camera with screen
- Light source
- Distending mechanism—Hysteroflator/Distention bag/Blood pressure cuff for inflation

- Normal saline
- Hysteroscope with operative sheath
- Hysteroscopic grasper
- Hysteroscopic scissors
- Transurethral resection (TUR) set
- Speculum/Vulsellum/Dilators.

DIAGNOSIS

Most of the times such retained foreign bodies remain asymptomatic and detected accidently as a work up for infertility or routine ultrasound assessment.

However, sometimes it may result in excessive vaginal discharge, intermenstrual bleeding or abnormal uterine bleeding. Some patients report to clinic with complaints of missing thread of intrauterine contraceptive device or pain lower abdomen due to the pelvic inflammatory disease (PID).

A routine ultrasound will usually detect an IUCD which is present in the uterus. An X-ray anteroposterior (AP) and lateral view to identify the location - intrauterine or extrauterine, could be done in a low resource setting if the ultrasound findings are not confirmatory. A 3D ultrasound is the best method to diagnose intracavitary lesions in uterus. MRI and CT scan are very rarely required if the other modalities fail to identify. Usually in earlier days such lost IUD could be removed by partly dilating cervix and probing cavity and pulling out with artery forcep but used to cause discomfort to patient. Hysteroscopy can be used both as diagnostic and therapeutic intervention in such cases.

TIMING OF PROCEDURE

The procedure should ideally be carried out postmenstrually so that the endometrium is thin and does not obstruct the view.

HYSTEROSCOPIC PROCEDURE

The procedure is carried out in a lithotomy position. If it is not an office procedure, suitable anesthesia would be given. A precursor diagnostic hysteroscopy may be done to confirm the site of the IUCD. The hysteroscope is then attached to an operative sheath. An alligator type grasping forcep is inserted through the operative channel. The jaws are opened to grip the thread which can then be pulled out to retrieve it.

If this fails, the lower point of shaft is held and IUCD is pulled gently to be removed with removal of operative sheath.

EMBEDDED INTRAUTERINE CONTRACEPTIVE DEVICES

Sometimes the foreign body is embedded deeply in the cavity and cannot be pulled out by the grasping forceps. In this case, the surgeon would need to use a scissor to cut around the myometrium to separate the IUCD. Rarely, a laparoscopic procedure may be required in case one suspects the IUCD has breached the serosa and may even be involving intraperitoneal structures, e.g. bowel.[9,10] One may also need to remove the IUCD piece meal and the retrieved parts are assembled outside to see for completeness of procedure.

RARE CASES

There have been cases in literature where a heavy foreign body like a broken tip of metal suction cannula has been retrieved by an innovative technique of using a laparoscopic tenaculum by the side of the hysteroscopic sheath.[11]

TIPS AND TRICKS

Maintaining good distension is the key to success in hysteroscopy. One of the best methods is to have the hysteroflator which gives a set pressure and the flow is controlled. The use of a nonreturning valve washer at the instrument channel of the hysteroscopic sheath reduces the loss of distension fluid while inserting and removing the instruments.

For Multiload IUCD, one may hold the foldable arms rather than the shaft as they may get splayed and stuck at the internal orifice of the uterus while retrieving it.

REFERENCES

1. Pushplata S, Devyani M, Pyari S, et al. Bizarre Foreign Objects in the Genital Tract-Our Experience and Review of literature. Open Journal of Obstetrics and Gynecology. 2014;427-31.
2. Sukru Y. Foreign body in vagina. J Turk Ger Gynecol Assoc. 2013;14(1):46-7.
3. Baral J, Rana A, Gurung G, et al. Rice grain in uterine cavity: Rare Presentations in Rural Nepalese Postmenopausal Framer with Uterovaginal Prolapse. J South Asian Feder Menopause Soc. 2014;2(2):79-82.
4. Bettocchi S, Di Spiezio Sardo A, Pinto L, et al. Hysteroscopic removal of gauze packing inadvertently sutured to the uterine cavity: report of 2 cases. J Minim Invasive Gynecol. 2009;16(1):88-91.
5. Tiufekchieva E . Corpus alienum in the uterus-Diagnostic and therapeuticHysteroscopy. Akush Ginekol (Sofia). 2007;46(5):28-32.
6. Osborne DF. Attempted abortion with retention of an intrauterine foreign body. Can Med Assoc J. 1964;90(7):494-5
7. Cetinkaya K, Kumtepe Y, Ingec M, et al . Minimally invasive approach to cases of lost intrauterine device: A 7 -year experience. Eur J Obstet Gynecol Reprod Biol. 2011;159(1):119-21.
8. Cepni I, Kumbak B, Ocal P, et al. Infertility due to intrauterine residual fetal bone fragments. J Clin Ultrasound. 2004;32(5):253-5.
9. Shah NH, et al. Intrauterine contraceptive device (IUCD) perforating bowel managed laparoscopically. JPGO. 2016; Volume 3 No.(12).
10. Shah NH, Paranjpe SH, Shah VN, et al. Laparoscopic retrieval of missing copper intrauterine device stuck to anterior abdominal wall presenting along with 8 weeks of pregnancy. JPGO. 2015;Volume 3 No.(1).
11. Shah NH, Paranjpe SH, Shah VN, et al. Innovative method of hysteroscopic retrieval of a broken metal suction cannula tip during MTP. JPGO. 2015;Volume 2 No.(12).

Chapter 8

Role of Hysteroscopy in Müllerian Anomaly

Rabi Narayan Satpathy

INTRODUCTION

Congenital anomalies of the female reproductive tract may involve the uterus, cervix, fallopian tubes or vagina. Depending on the specific defect, a woman's obstetric and gynecologic health may be adversely affected. Uterine anomalies are the most common of the müllerian anomalies, but the true incidence is not known since many women are asymptomatic and sensitive imaging modalities have only recently become available.[1] Uterine anomalies are associated with both normal and adverse reproductive outcomes. They occur in approximately 3–4% of infertile women, 5–10% of women with recurrent early pregnancy loss and 25% of women with late first or second trimester pregnancy loss or preterm delivery.[2] Overall, uterine anomalies are associated with difficulty maintaining a pregnancy. The proper management of müllerian anomalies is controversial.

EMBRYOLOGY

Normal development of the female reproductive tract requires a complex series of events: müllerian duct elongation, fusion, canalization and septal resorption. Failure of any part of this process can result in congenital anomaly. Müllerian development occurs in close association with development of the urinary tract. So anomalies of the kidney and ureter are commonly identified in females with müllerian anomalies. Gonadal development occurs as a separate process, therefore, women with müllerian anomalies usually have normal ovaries and ovarian hormone production.

The paired müllerian ducts are identifiable by 6th week of development and arise from coelomic epithelium along the lateral walls of the urogenital ridge. These solid tissue structures elongate caudally, cross the Wolffian ducts medially and fuse in the midline to form the primitive uterovaginal canal. By 10th week, the caudal end of the fused müllerian ducts connects with the urogenital sinus. Next internal canalization of the müllerian ducts occurs resulting in two channels divided by a septum. The septum is subsequently resorbed in the caudal to cephalad direction and is completed by 20th week.

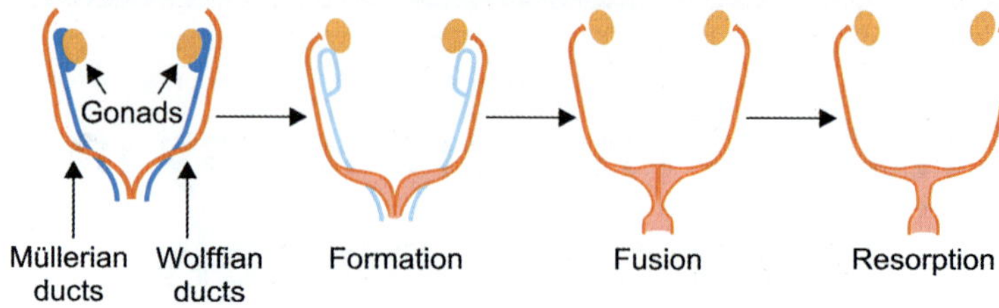

Fig. 1: Development of the female reproductive tract.

The fused caudal portion of the müllerian ducts becomes the uterus and upper vagina and the unfused cephalad portion becomes the fallopian tubes (Fig. 1).

PATHOPHYSIOLOGY

Congenital anomalies of the female reproductive tract are typically classified into three main categories: (1) agenesis and hypoplasia, (2) lateral fusion defects, and (3) vertical fusion defects. A fourth group is composed of women exposed to diethylstilbestrol (DES) in-utero. Agenesis and hypoplasia can occur with any or multiple müllerian structures. Lateral fusion defects occur due to failure of migration of one müllerian duct or failure of absorption of the intervening septum between the ducts. This is the most common category of müllerian defect and can result in symmetric or asymmetric and non-obstructed or obstructed structures. Vertical fusion defects result from abnormal fusion of the müllerian ducts with the urogenital sinus or problems with vaginal canalization.[3] These lesions can cause menstrual flow obstruction.

CLASSIFICATION

There is no universally accepted standard classification for congenital anomalies of the female reproductive tract. In 1988, the American Fertility Society or the American Society for Reproductive Medicine created a classification system that focuses on the major categories of uterine anomalies.[4]

- Class I: Uterine hypoplasia/agenesis
- Class II: Unicornuate uterus
- Class III: Uterus didelphys
- Class IV: Bicornuate uterus
  - Complete: When the indentation produced in the fundic region is deep, thus indicating that fusion failed from the level of the cervical region.
  - Incomplete: When the division is higher, not extending to the level of the cervix, indicated by the shallower indentation in the contour of the region of the uterine fundus.
- Class V: Septate uterus
  - Complete: When the septum extends into the internal cervical ostium, possibly including the cervical canal and divides the cervix into two tunneled cavities.

  - Partial: When the septum does not divide the uterine cavity along its entire length and circulation exists between the two chambers.
- Class VI: Arcuate uterus
- Class VII: T-shaped uterus resulting from the use of DES.

CLINICAL FEATURES

Although many women with müllerian anomalies are asymptomatic, several gynecologic signs and symptoms are associated with specific anomalies. Women may present with cyclic or noncyclic pelvic pain and dysmenorrhea suggestive of an obstructive anomaly, retrograde menstruation and endometriosis.[5] Primary amenorrhea with pelvic pain or back pain or a pelvic mass is concerning for a transverse vaginal septum or an imperforate hymen. Müllerian agenesis presents with primary amenorrhea. Abnormal uterine bleeding may occur with a septate uterus or a partial or microperforate obstruction.

Of all müllerian anomalies, those involving the uterus are most commonly implicated in poor obstetric outcomes. Uterine anomalies are associated with diminished cavity size, insufficient musculature, impaired ability to distend, abnormal myometrial and cervical function, inadequate vascularity and abnormal endometrial development. These abnormalities of space, vascular supply and associated local defects contribute to increased rates of recurrent pregnancy loss, preterm delivery and malpresentation. Intrauterine growth restriction is similarly attributed to abnormal vascularization and a smaller uterine cavity.[6] Other associated obstetrical complications include cervical incompetence, pregnancy induced hypertension (due to renal anomalies) and antepartum or postpartum bleeding.

DIAGNOSIS

Several radiologic techniques are useful for evaluating congenital anomalies of the female reproductive tract. Modalities employed include hysteroscopy, hysterosalpingogram (HSG), ultrasonography and magnetic resonance imaging (MRI). Each imaging technique has inherent strengths and limitations. Therefore a combination of several techniques may best evaluate a particular abnormality.

Diagnostic Hysteroscopy

Hysteroscopy is the visualization of uterine cavity by endoscopy through the cervix. It allows diagnosis of any uterine anomaly, if present, and its surgical management at same time. Previously laparotomy used to be performed for diagnosis and management of müllerian anomaly. It was a time consuming procedure. After the use of hysteroscopy, the diagnosis and treatment of uterine anomaly is very much simplified.

HSG is also used to diagnose any müllerian anomaly. It helps to assess the patency of fallopian tubes and can provide further information about the contour of the endometrial cavity and the presence of any complex communications. Definitive diagnosis of a uterine abnormality requires assessment of the external uterine contour and this is poorly defined by HSG. The HSG correctly diagnoses 55% of septate and bicornuate uteri and the addition of ultrasonography improves this result to 90%.[7]

Ultrasonography effectively evaluates the internal and external uterine contour, detects a pelvic mass, hematometra or hematocolpos, confirms the presence of ovaries and assesses the kidneys. Study during the secretory phase of the menstrual cycle provides better visualization of the endometrium and thus the internal uterine contour.

Sonohysterography can further delineate the intracavitary space and internal and external uterine contours. Three-dimensional ultrasonography is a highly accurate imaging modality that provides thorough views of the pelvic anatomy and detailed visualization of the uterus. This is a very reliable method for evaluating müllerian anomalies.[8]

MRI is considered the gold standard technique for diagnosing müllerian anomalies and is both sensitive and specific. This modality provides excellent delineation of internal and external uterine contours. MRI can distinguish between bicornuate, didelphic and septate uteri and can determine the extent of a uterine or vaginal septum. Furthermore, MRI can identify a rudimentary uterine horn and determine if functional endometrium is present.[9]

Saravelos in 2008 reviewed the medical literature in order to assess the diagnostic accuracy of different methodologies and estimate the prevalence of congenital uterine anomalies in women with infertility and recurrent miscarriage. They concluded that the most accurate diagnostic procedures were combined hysteroscopy and laparoscopy, sonohysterography and possibly three-dimensional ultrasound.[10] Despite the fact that the gold standard in the diagnosis of uterine anomalies is the combined application of laparoscopy and hysteroscopy, one has to bear in mind that it is mainly based on the subjective impression of the clinician performing them.

Anomalies of the urinary tract are frequently seen with müllerian anomalies. Thus appropriate urinary tract imaging is necessary. Upper urinary tract abnormalities include renal anomalies such as a horseshoe kidney or pelvic kidney or renal agenesis, duplication of the collecting system and ectopic ureters. In the setting of an obstructive müllerian defect such as a noncommunicating uterine horn or an obstructed hemivagina, ipsilateral renal agenesis is commonly seen. Over 50% of cases, renal agenesis is predictive of a müllerian anomaly.[11] Recommended imaging techniques for the urinary tract are an intravenous pyelogram (IVP), renal ultrasound or a computed tomography (CT) scan.

Therapeutic Hysteroscopy

Due to the availability of sophisticated imaging techniques, diagnostic surgical procedures such as an examination under anesthesia, vaginoscopy, hysteroscopy and laparoscopy are rarely necessary to diagnose müllerian anomalies. But historically, laparoscopy and hysteroscopy were the gold standard for evaluating the contour of the uterine fundus and assigning the proper classification to a uterine anomaly. Currently surgery for müllerian anomalies is indicated for women with pelvic pain, endometriosis, obstructive anomalies and poor obstetric outcomes. Prior to performing surgery, it is important to exclude extrauterine factors which may cause pregnancy loss. The goals of surgery include treatment of pelvic pain, restoration of pelvic anatomy and uterine architecture and preservation of fertility.

Transcervical Resection of the Septum

In cases of uterine septum, the resection should be performed hysteroscopically in order to improve the reproductive prognosis for the patient by decreasing the incidence of miscarriage, premature delivery and infertility. This is known as *transcervical resection of septum (TCRS)*. The advantages of hysteroscopy include the shorter duration of surgery, smaller blood loss, lower costs, reduced morbidity and shorter hospital stay, compared with abdominal surgery. In cases of complete uterine septum, resection of the cervical septum may be related to cervical incompetence and secondary infertility.[12] Concomitant laparoscopy enables evaluation of the pelvis and external uterine contour and guides the extent of septum resection. Traditionally the cervical portion of a complete septum is left intact due to the risk of cervical incompetence, but a recent small randomized study demonstrated that resection of the cervical septum is associated with a less complicated surgical procedure and equivalent reproductive outcomes.[13]

Hysteroscopic Metroplasty

Hysteroscopic metroplasty in women with recurrent miscarriage and a septate uterus is being performed to improve reproductive outcomes. However, only noncontrolled studies suggesting a positive effect on pregnancy outcomes have been performed so far. These studies are biased due to the fact that the participants with recurrent miscarriage treated by hysteroscopic metroplasty served as their own controls. No randomized controlled trial evaluating the effectiveness and possible complications of hysteroscopic metroplasty has been published so far. The Strassman metroplasty is a better option. It achieves unification of two endometrial cavities in a divided uterus (bicornuate or didelphys) and is associated with a live birth rate greater than 80%. But several experts believe that existing data do not support repair of a didelphic uterus to improve pregnancy outcome.[14]

Hysteroscopic Intrauterine Devices Insertion

Intrauterine devices are postsurgical alternatives for minimizing formation of uterine adherences or synechiae. The follow-up in these cases includes hysteroscopy 1–3 months after the initial surgery.

Uterovaginal Anastomosis

Most cervical abnormalities accompany vaginal or uterine anomalies. The cervical anomalies include agenesis, atresia, abnormal length or width, obstruction and hypertrophy. Cervical atresia is a rare anomaly. These women can present with primary amenorrhea and cyclic pelvic pain due to hematometra and retrograde menstruation. Successful pregnancies have occurred after uterovaginal anastomosis for cervical atresia.[15] Surgical correction of obstructive cervical anomalies rarely results in a patent passage and is associated with a high risk of ascending infection.

Resection of Vaginal Septum

Each vaginal anomaly requires careful assessment of pelvic anatomy to make the correct diagnosis and surgical repair is necessary in the presence of an obstructive anomaly. A transverse vaginal septum results from failure of fusion between the müllerian ducts and the urogenital sinus or abnormal vaginal canalization and requires excision of the septum and vaginal anastomosis. A longitudinal vaginal septum may cause dyspareunia, difficulty with tampon placement or obstructed labor and should be excised. An imperforate hymen occurs due to incomplete degeneration of the central portion of the hymen and requires excision of the excess hymenal tissue.

Role of Laparoscopy

The unicornuate uterus is an uncommon anomaly which may be associated with relatively poor reproductive outcome depending on a number of factors such as variations in the vascular contribution from the uterine artery and ovarian artery of the contralateral side, extent of the reduction of muscular mass, degree of cervical incompetence and presence of coexistent pelvic disease such as endometriosis. The rudimentary horn can be removed by laparoscopic surgery. It is also used for diagnosis of cervical agenesis and hypoplastic uterus in Mayer-Rokitansky-Küster-Hauser (MRKH) syndrome. Neovaginoplasty procedure is done in cases of MRKH with vaginal agenesis. In many women the malformation results in obstruction of the outflow tract and retrograde menstruation, thereby facilitating the development of endometriosis. During laparoscopy, this diagnosis may be confirmed and the endometrial foci may be resected out.

CONCLUSION

Müllerian anomalies consist of a wide range of defects that may vary from patient to patient. Therefore their management must be individualized taking anatomical and clinical characteristics into consideration as well as the patient's wishes. Although these anomalies are relatively uncommon, they can significantly impact reproductive outcomes. A high index of suspicion is warranted in adolescents and reproductive age women with pelvic pain, dysmenorrhea, abnormal bleeding, recurrent pregnancy loss or preterm delivery. Detailed pelvic imaging with modalities such as HSG, ultrasonography, hysteroscopy and MRI is necessary as well as evaluation of the urinary tract as indicated.

When a müllerian anomaly is identified, the woman should be counseled about reproductive prognosis, pregnancy outcomes and evidence-based management. Many of these women can have normal reproductive outcomes, but intervention is recommended in the event of poor obstetric outcomes. Moreover, due to the ease and low morbidity associated with septal resection and hysteroscopic metroplasty, these procedures should be considered in infertile women with a septate uterus prior to advanced fertility treatment. The diagnosis and classification of müllerian anomalies are facilitated by the availability of excellent imaging modalities, hence current data on reproductive outcomes with uterine anomalies should be assessed.

REFERENCES

1. Lin PC, Bhatnagar KP, Nettleton GS, et al. Female genital anomalies affecting reproduction. Fertil Steril. 2002;78:899-915.
2. Raga F, Bauset C, Remohi J. Reproductive impact of congenital mullerian anomalies. Hum Reprod. 1997;12:2277-81.
3. Iverson RE, DeCherney AH, Laufer MR, et al. Clinical manifestations and diagnosis of congenital anomalies of the uterus. Netherlands: Wolters Kluwer; 2007.
4. The American Fertility Society classifications of adnexal adhesions, distal tubal occlusion, tubal occlusion secondary to tubal ligation, tubal pregnancies, mullerian anomalies and intrauterine adhesions. Fertil Steril. 1988;49:944-55.
5. Sanfilippo JS, Wakim NG, Schikler KN, et al. Endometriosis in association with uterine anomaly. Am J Obstet Gynecol. 2016; 154:39-43.
6. Andrews MC, Jones HW Jr. Impaired reproductive performance of the anomalous uterus: intrauterine growth retardation, infertility, and recurrent abortion in five cases. Am J Obstet Gynecol. 1982;144:173-6.
7. Troiano RN, McCarthy SM. Mullerian duct anomalies: imaging and clinical issues. Radiology. 2004;233:19-34.
8. Goldberg JM, Falcone T, Attaran M. Ultrasonographic evaluation of uterine abnormalities noted on hysterosalpingography. Hum Reprod. 2007;12:2151-3.
9. Pellerito JS, McCarthy SM, Doyle MB, et al. Diagnosis of uterine anomalies: relative accuracy of MR imaging, vaginal sonography and hysterosalpingography. Radiology. 1992;183:795-800.
10. Saravelos SH, Cocksedge KH, Li TC. Prevalence and diagnosis of congenital uterine anomalies in women with reproductive failure: a critical appraisal. Hum Reprod Update. 2008;14(5):415-29.
11. Jayasinghe Y, Rane A, Stalewski H, et al. The presentation and early diagnosis of the rudimentary uterine horn. Obst Gynecol. 2005;105:1456-67.
12. Bakas P, Gregoriou O, Hassiakos D, et al. Hysteroscopic resection of uterine septum and reproductive outcome in women with unexplained infertility. Gynecol Obstet Invest. 2012;73(4):321-5.
13. Parsanezhad ME, Alborzi S, Zarei A. Hysteroscopic metroplasty of the complete uterine septum, duplicate cervi and vaginal septum. Fertil Steril. 2006;85:1473-7.
14. Kowalik CR, Goddijn M, Emanuel MH, et al. Metroplasty versus expectant management for women with recurrent miscarriage and a septate uterus. Cochrane Database Syst Rev. 2011;(6):CD008576.
15. Deffarges JV, Haddad B, Musset R, et al. Utero-vaginal anastomosis in women with uterine cervix atresia: long -term follow- up and reproductive performance: a study of 18 cases. Hum Reprod. 2001;16:1722.

Chapter 9

Hysteroscopic Myomectomy

Malvika Sabharwal

INTRODUCTION

Leiomyomas are the most common tumors of the uterus. The incidence of leiomyosarcoma is of 0.1%. The complaints may be abnormal uterine bleeding (AUB), infertility, recurrent pregnancy loss (RPL), dysmenorrhea, abdominal discomfort and sensation of weight in the pelvis.[1]

All fibroids need not to be operated, even the submucous. Only symptomatic fibroid causing infertility, RPL or AUB need to be dealt with. Transvaginal sonography (TVS) indicates the number, size and the location of fibroids and the possibility of an intramural component of the submucous fibroid. Besides, it also investigates the uterine adnexa.[2] Hysteroscopy confirms the findings (Fig. 1). Hysterosonography adds an important data to preoperative investigation of submucous fibroid showing the depth of fibroid and distance of free myometrium.[3] Magnetic resonance imaging (MRI) of the pelvis may help in the diagnosis of other causes of AUB, especially adenomyosis.[4] Fibroid and adenomyosis coexist in almost 30% of the cases.

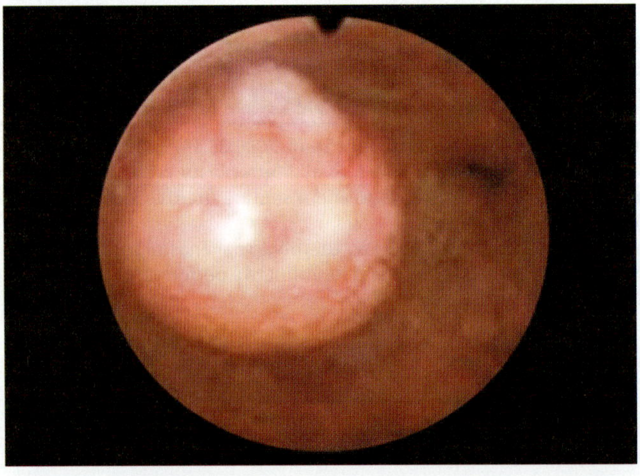

Fig. 1: Hysteroscopic image showing the submucous fibroid.

CLASSIFICATION

The most used classification system is the European Society for Gynaecological Endoscopy (ESGE) that has as evaluation factor for the degree of the penetration of the submucous fibroid into the myometrium.[5] This classification is simple and objective and is divided in various levels (Fig. 2):

- Level 0 - myomas that are completely within the uterine cavity
- Level 1 - more than 50% of the nodule is in the uterine cavity
- Level 2 - more than 50% of the fibroid is within the myometrium.

In 2005, Lasmar et al. published a new classification of submucous fibroid, called "STEP-W" classification (Table 1). The anterior and posterior wall fibroid gets a score 0.

Score Group Suggested Treatment Process

- 0-4 (I) Low complexity hysteroscopic myomectomy
- 5-6 (II) Complex hysteroscopic myomectomy, consider preparing with gonadotropin-releasing hormone (GnRH) analog and/or 2-stage surgery
- 7-9 (III) Recommend an alternative non-hysteroscopic technique.

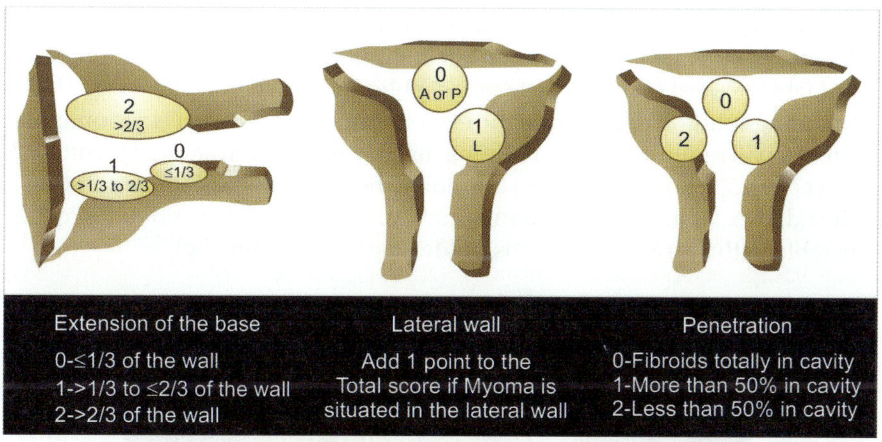

Fig. 2: Score based evaluation of myoma.

Table 1: Parameters used to classify the submucous myoma.

	Size	*Topography*	*Extension*	*Penetration*	*Lateral wall*
0	= 2 cm	Lower	= 1/3	0	+1
1	> 2–5 cm	Medium	1/3 – 2/3	= 50%	+1
2		Upper	> 2/3	> 50%	+1
Score		+	+	+	+

Preoperative Preparation

The GnRH analogues may be used prior to hysteroscopy to reduce the size of the myoma and the uterus at preoperative preparation. It decreases the myoma size, vascularity and consequently fluid absorption is less.[6] However, for some authors the use of analogues before surgery would be associated with a greater recurrence of fibroids and a high risk of uterine perforation.[7] There is no consensus regarding the same, thus it should be reserved for well selected patients. The hysteroscopic myomectomy may also be indicated to patients that have contraindications to undergo major surgery. Uterine artery embolization has also been mentioned which interrupts metrorrhagia and reduces fibroid vascularization allowing big nodules to be removed with very little risk of intravasation and bleeding.

SURGICAL TECHNIQUES

Resectoscopy

This is the most commonly employed approach. The resectoscope is the instrument that resects under direct and constant visual control. The sheath has an outer diameter of 7–9 mm, and includes both inflow and outflow ports for distending media. If surgical debris or the so-called 'chips' blocks the operative field, the resectoscope can be removed while the sheath is left in place. This allows for removal of large tissue while maintaining cervical dilatation. It has a straight-forward or a slightly forward-oblique telescope 12/30° (Fig. 3). The distending solution depends on the electrosurgical system, if it is a monopolar system it will require a nonconducting distending solution such as sorbitol 5% or glycine 1.5%, but if the system is bipolar, the use of normal saline solution is allowed. If excessive intravasation occurs, the isotonic fluid overload is readily treatable with diuretics (e.g. furosemide 20 mg intravenously).

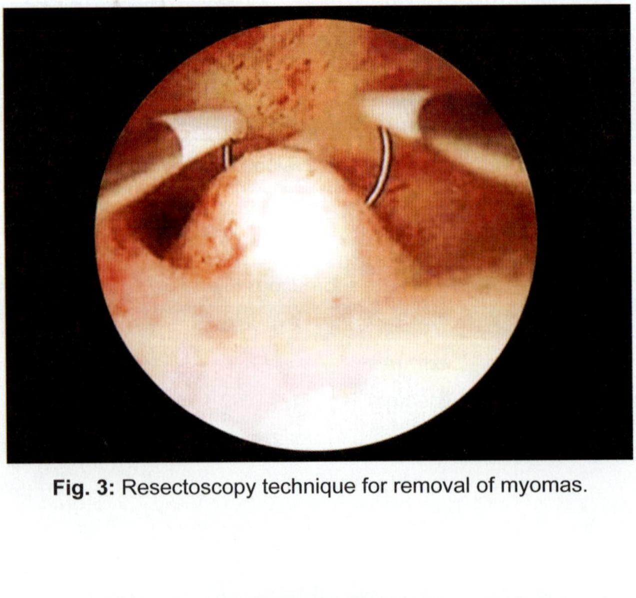

Fig. 3: Resectoscopy technique for removal of myomas.

Generally, most protocols and guidelines mention about 2,500 mL as the upper limit of saline intravasation. The use of a bipolar set of instruments, in which both electrodes are introduced into the thermal loop, would be much safer. The diameters of thermal loops for bipolar resectoscopes are usually smaller than loops for a monopolar instrument with the same outer diameter, thus increasing the time required for resection.[1] Although bipolar techniques are less hazardous because of intravasation and electrolyte blood-imbalances, more gas-bubbles may hamper visualization, and gas-emboli might cause spasms in the lung capillaries, potentially disturbing gas diffusion in the lungs. The removal of type-0 and type-1 lesions is generally straightforward. It consist of repeated and progressive passages of the cutting loop beyond the myoma, with cutting only taking place during the backward or return movement of the loop. Excision usually begins from the top of the fibroid, progressing in a uniform way towards the base. The surgery is considered finished when the fasciculate structure of the myometrium is visualized. Although in some cases they can be removed by one-step procedure, but most of the surgeons prefer to remove this kind of myomas through a two-step procedure. For type 1 and type 2 there is a high risk of damage of the healthy myometrium during electrosurgery, both by cutting and by thermal damage.

Morcellator

Currently, we can find in the market three different hysteroscopic morcellators, the Truclear (Smith and Nephew, Andover MA, USA), the MyoSure by Hologic (Bedford MA, USA) and another company that recently introduced an alternative device is Storz (Tuttlingen, Germany). The system uses no electrocoagulation, and there is no lateral thermal or electrical energy spread. Hemostasis occurs by spontaneous myometrial contraction. The removed tissue is available for pathology analysis. Saline solution is used for distension

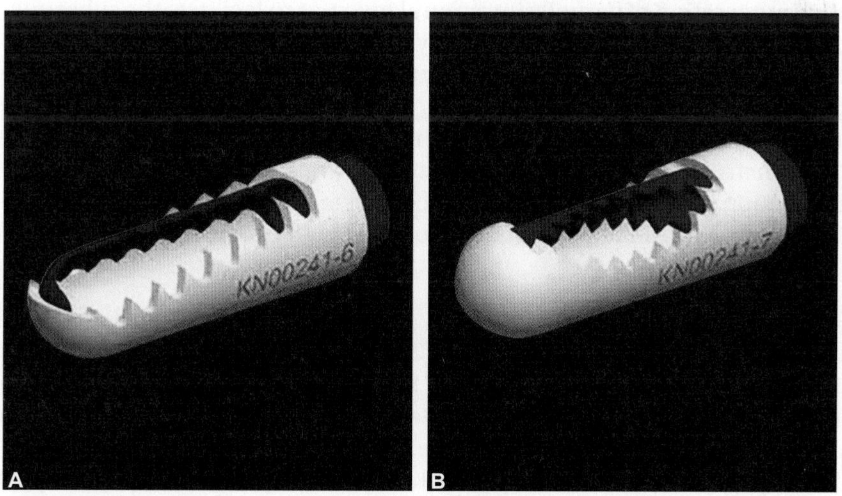

Fig. 4: Morcellator.

and irrigation. Although promising at this moment the level of evidence for the use of hysteroscopic morcellator for submucous fibroids is limited, more trials are needed.

Vaporization

Although argon, krypton and neodymium-doped yttrium-aluminum garnet (Nd:YAG) lasers have all been successfully used, only the latter has found widespread application in hysteroscopic surgery,[8] being very popular in the late 1980s and early 1990s. Two techniques 'touch' and 'non-touch' may be used in hysteroscopic Nd:YAG laser surgery for fibroids of 2 cm or less.[9,10] In the former, the laser fiber is in contact with the surface to be treated coagulating first the surface vessels and then the fiber is dragged repetitiously over the fibroid until it is flattened, whereas in the latter it is separated from it by a few millimeters. In hysteroscopic myomectomy both techniques were used.[8] This technique is not in use because of the high cost.

Hysteroscopic outpatient laser applications (HoLA by Biolitec, Germany), is a diode laser with a power of 120 W using a Myofiber of 9 Fr for submucous myoma vaporization in an office setting. Although it is effective for fibroid tissue vaporization but it has some limitations:

- The fiber diameter requires a 6.3 mm hysteroscope that is not well tolerated by most of the patients without anesthesia
- The power of 120 W is necessary in order to achieve tissue vaporization; the heat created by the laser is painful for the patient when it is used near the myometrium
- Lack of specimens for histopathology analysis
- The level of evidence for the use of diode laser for fibroids vaporization is limited and more trials are needed.
- Distension of the uterine cavity was obtained with saline solution.

In 2009, Bettocchi et al. described a new hysteroscopic technique for the office preparation of partially intramural myomas to facilitate the subsequent scheduled resectoscopic myomectomy. The procedure consists of an incision of the endometrial mucosa and the pseudocapsule covering the myoma aimed at facilitating protrusion of the intramural portion of the myoma into the uterine cavity as a preliminary step for inpatient resectoscopic surgery after two menstrual cycles. The myoma is transformed from G2 or G1 to G0 and enucleation is facilitated. The result is complete enucleation without injury to the uterine wall and reduced risks associated with classic slicing.

Enucleation in Toto

A technique described by Litta et al. in 2003, for the treatment of myomas with high intramural involvement (G1-G2), that favors the intracavitary protrusion of the myoma ensuring safe removal while minimizing damage to the surrounding myometrium. This is a safe technique that enables transformation of the myoma from G2 to G0, allowing the surgeon to perform a completely safe myomectomy within the uterine cavity. This results in reduction of perforation of the uterine wall.

Cold Loop Myomectomy

The technique, developed by Mazzon, is characterized by a sequence of three different operating steps:

1. Excision of the intracavitary component of the fibroid: This is carried out with the usual technique of resectoscope slicing.
2. Enucleation of the intramural component of the fibroid: Once the cleavage plane is identified, the usual cutting loop of the resectoscope is substituted by a suitable blunt dissection cold loop (mechanical loops of Mazzon; Karl Storz, Tuttlingen, Germany). During the entire phase of enucleation, electric energy must not be used in the thickness of the wall, and the loop must be used 'cold' or in a mechanical way.
3. Excision of the intramural component using an angled cutting loop. Versapoint (bipolar energy) and Mechanical Instruments (scissors and forceps) are used in office setting hysteroscopy. In some cases of small myomas, it is possible to achieve enucleation. According to Bettocchi et al, it is feasible to operate this way, myoma up to 20 mm using a 5 Fr bipolar electrode.

COMPLICATIONS OF HYSTEROSCOPY

Laceration of the uterine cervix and uterine perforation are two of the most frequent complications, mainly when the use of GnRH analog precede the procedure, causing atrophy and difficulty of cervical dilation with Hegar dilator. When uterine perforation occurred with the use of electric current, either mono or bipolar, it is necessary to investigate the abdominal cavity to investigate injuries on the bladder or bowel. The bladder injury has an earlier diagnosis, as hematuria is immediately present. At this moment, cystoscopy is performed. The bowel loop injuries may not be noticed in most of the cases in the hysteroscopic surgeries. It does not have a sign or immediate symptom, and peritonitis is the late symptomatology. Uterine perforation at hysteroscopic surgeries should be suspected when it is difficult to maintain the intrauterine pressure and/or when there is a very fast negative hydric balance. In these cases of fast escape of fluid distension medium, it is mandatory to interrupt the procedure and investigate the bladder, and in some cases the abdominal and pelvic cavity by laparoscopy or laparotomy. As the fibroid has large caliber vessels, bleeding is an important issue. Coagulation should be performed in all arterial and venous vessels with large caliber. Inserting a Foley catheter with a distending balloon for 6 to 12 hours is an option to control diffuse bleeding, as extended coagulation would lead to major injuries. Although some authors[11] suggested that perioperative oxytocin may decrease bleeding during myomectomy. Cochrane recent review[12] does not depict effective decrease of bleeding with the use of misoprostol, oxytocin, tourniquet, morcellation, vasopressin and epinephrine with bupivacaine. Fluid absorption may occur in a very fast way, which could cause intravasation and death. Rigorous control of hydric balance is important, thus it is necessary to be careful from 1 L of negative balance, and it should not reach 2 L in saline media. Infection is infrequent in hysteroscopic surgeries, with greater incidences in myomectomy. The presence of remnants facilitates the infectious process, leading to the formation of hematometra. Prophylactic antibiotic therapy is indicated in this procedure. Gas embolization is rare, but fatal. Some late complications happen such as synechia and mainly in the area of large resections. Some authors have described that the incidence of synechiae after hysteroscopic myomectomy vary from 1–13%.

FINAL CONSIDERATIONS

Hysteroscopic myomectomy is the best way to treat intracavitary uterine disease and potentially preserve its structure. Submucous fibroid excision by hysteroscopy has reduced morbidity, length of hospital stay and postoperative pain, besides it is more economical, with fast recovery and return to daily activities and earlier return to sexual activity than laproscopic myomectomy/hysterectomy.

REFERENCES

1. Indman P. Hysteroscopic treatment of submucous myomas. Clinical Obstetrics and Gynaecology. 2006;49(4):811-20.
2. Bronz L, Suter T, Rusca T. The value of transvaginal sonography with and without saline instillation in the diagnosis of uterine pathology in pre and post menopausal women with abnormal bleeding or suspect sonographic findings. Ultrasound Obstet Gynaecol. 1997;9(1): 53-8.
3. Bernard JP, Lecuru F, Darles C, et al. Saline contrast sonohysterography as first line investigation for women with uterine bleeding. Ultrasound Obstet Gynaecol. 1997;110(10):121-5.
4. Werner H, Brandão A, Daltro P. Ressonância magnética em Obstetrícia e Ginecologia. 1ª edição, Revinter 2003.
5. Wamsteker K, Emanuel MH, deKruif JH. Transcervical hysteroscopic resection of submucous fibroids for abnormal uterine bleeding: Results regarding degree of intramural extension. Obstet Gynecol. 1993;82(5):736-40.
6. Falcone T, Gustilo AM. Minimally invasive surgery for mass lesions. Clin Obstet Gynecol. 2005; 48(2): 353-60.
7. Murakami T, Tamura M, Ozawa Y, et al. Safe techniques in surgery for hysteroscopic myomectomy. J Obstet Gynaecol Res. 2005;31(3):216-23.
8. Ubaldi F, Tournaye H, Camus M, et al. Fertility after hysteroscopic myomectomy. Hum Reprod Update. 1995;88(1):81-90.
9. Goldrath MH, Fuller TA, Segal S. Laser photovaporization of endometrium for the treatment of menorrhagia. Am J Obstet Gynecol. 1981;140(1):14-19.
10. Loffer FD. Hysteroscopic endometrial ablation with the Nd:Yag laser using a nontouch technique. Obstet Gynecol.1987;69(4):679-82.
11. Wang CJ, Lee CL, Yuen LT, et al. Oxytocin infusion in laparoscopic myomectomy may decrease operative blood loss. J Minim Invasive Gynecol. 2007;14(2):184-8.
12. Kongnyuiy J, Wiysonge S. Interventions to reduce haemorrhage during myomectomy for fibroids. Cochrane Database Syst Rev. 2011;9(11):CD005355.

Chapter 10

Transcervical Resection of Uterine Septum

Parul Kotdawala

INTRODUCTION

Uterine septum is the commonest mullerian developmental anomaly where the uterine cavity is divided vertically by a myometrial segment. It is the mullerian malformation with the highest incidence of reproductive complications and poor reproductive outcomes like increased risk of spontaneous abortion and preterm delivery. There are two kinds of uterine septum starting from the fundus of the uterus. If it extends up to the internal os of the cervix, it is classified as a complete septum and if it does not, it is a partial septum (Fig. 1).

EMBRYOLOGICAL DEVELOPMENT OF UTERUS

To understand the uterine septum, one needs to know the normal development of the uterus from the mullerian ducts. Any disturbance in the mechanism by which the mullerian ducts fuse to form a single cervix, uterus and upper vagina

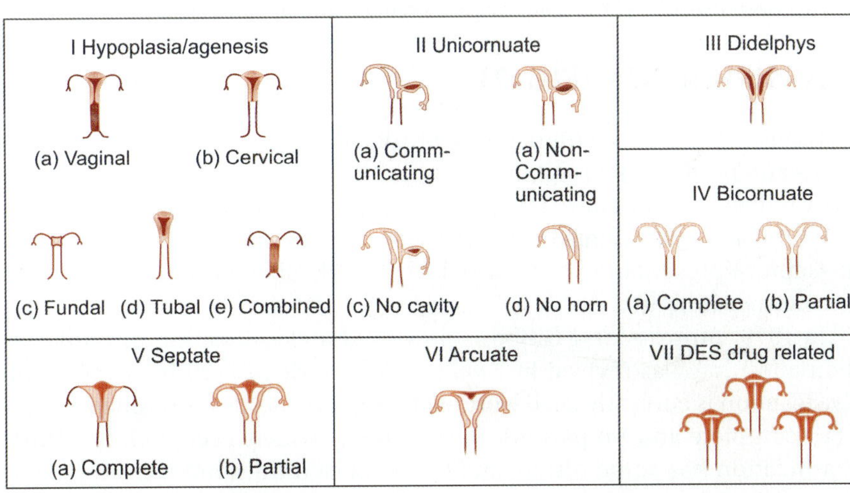

Fig. 1: Classification of uterine cavity septal developmental anomalies.

through the process of differentiation, migration, fusion and canalization leads to the development of mullerian duct anomaly.

The paired mullerian ducts arise as longitudinal invaginations of celomic epithelium on the outer side of the urogenital ridge. This process of differentiation occurs in the 6th week of pregnancy. After this 1st phase the mullerian ducts grow caudally, lateral to the mesonephric ducts. They then cross the ridge medially and fuse with each other. This fused ducts solidify and extend caudally to create the uterine primordium by around 9th week. At the same time the invagination of the urogenital sinus is reached. Later at 10th week of pregnancy the canalization of the fused mullerian ducts take place, resulting in 2 channels with a septum between them.

Finally, the process concludes with the resorption of this septum in a caudal to cephalad direction, which is completed around 9-10th week resulting in a single uterus, cervix, upper vagina and two fallopian tubes - the uppermost parts of the mesonephric ducts.

So a septate uterus is the result of failure of resorption of the medial septum that range from complete or partial. The uterine septum regresses by the process of apoptosis. The presence of BIC-2 protein is implicated in this apoptosis mechanism. The absence of BIC-2 in the embryo and uterine septum may indicate a lack of protection from apoptosis in this area.[1] However, there are various other studies which have identified several genes that can implicate in the development of uterine malformations.[2,3]

INCIDENCE

Chang reported in his 94 observational studies comprising 89,861 women, that the prevalence of uterine anomalies was 5.5% in unselected population, 8% in infertile women, 13.3% in those with history of miscarriage and infertility.[4] The most common uterine anomaly diagnosed in the unselected population was arcuate uterus (3.9%) followed by septate uterus (2.3%).

CLASSIFICATION (FIG. 2)

Classically the septate uterus has been divided into two types: complete septate uterus and partial or subseptate uterus. In the complete septum, the uterine cavity is divided in its entire length by the septum, which reaches the internal os. While in the subseptate uterus, the septum does not reach the internal os. The septum presentations are varied with markedly different length, width and internal structure.

In 1979, Buttram and Gibbons proposed a classification in mullerian anomalies that was revised in 1988 by the American Fertility Society, this classification is currently used worldwide. Septate uterus is classified as class V (Va complete and Vb partial). Despite being widely accepted, the ASRM classification has some disadvantages because it does not classify vaginal anomalies and is unable to classify uteri with multiple anomalies.[5,6]

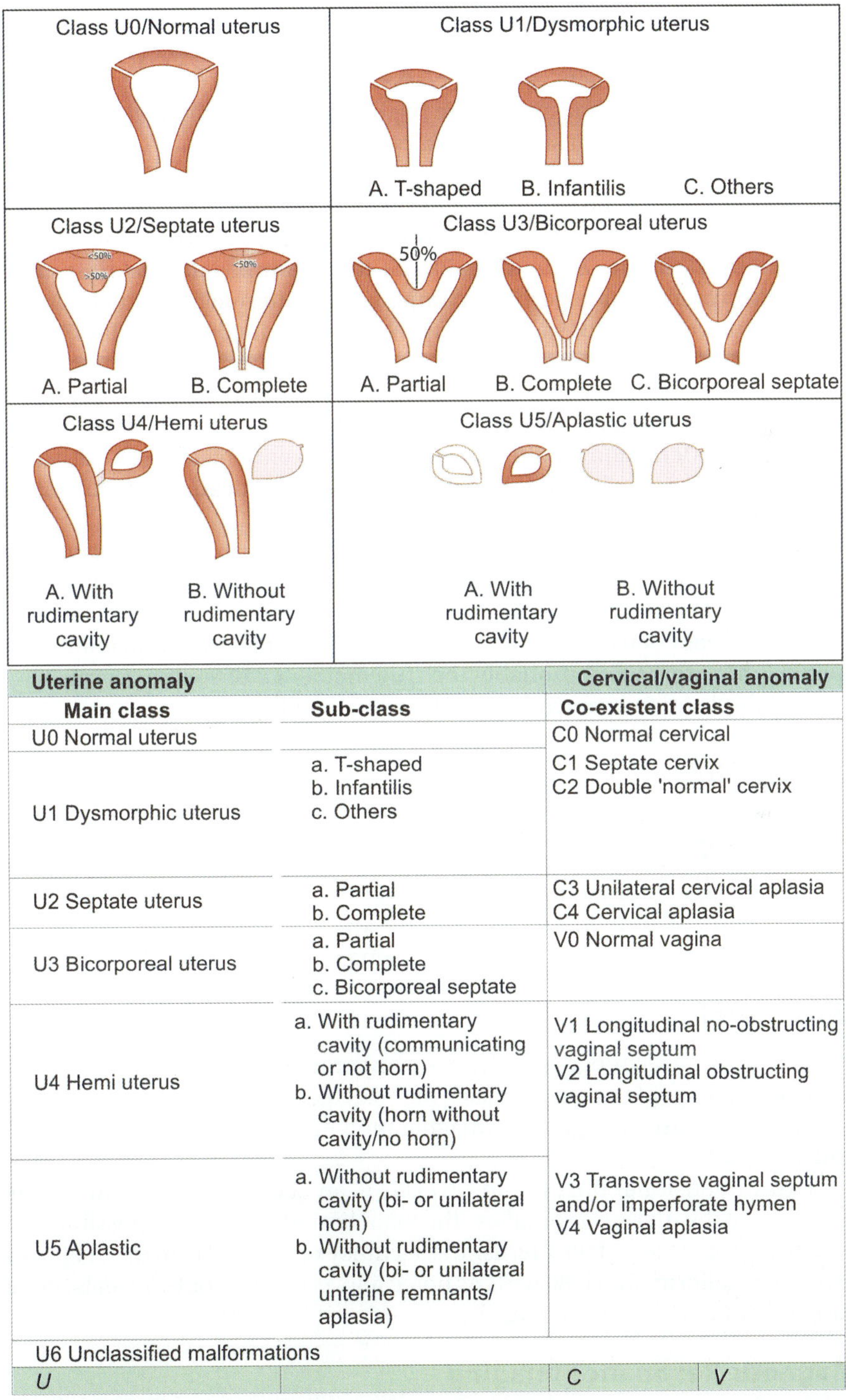

Uterine anomaly		Cervical/vaginal anomaly
Main class	**Sub-class**	**Co-existent class**
U0 Normal uterus		C0 Normal cervical
U1 Dysmorphic uterus	a. T-shaped b. Infantilis c. Others	C1 Septate cervix C2 Double 'normal' cervix
U2 Septate uterus	a. Partial b. Complete	C3 Unilateral cervical aplasia C4 Cervical aplasia
U3 Bicorporeal uterus	a. Partial b. Complete c. Bicorporeal septate	V0 Normal vagina
U4 Hemi uterus	a. With rudimentary cavity (communicating or not horn) b. Without rudimentary cavity (horn without cavity/no horn)	V1 Longitudinal no-obstructing vaginal septum V2 Longitudinal obstructing vaginal septum
U5 Aplastic	a. Without rudimentary cavity (bi- or unilateral horn) b. Without rudimentary cavity (bi- or unilateral unterine remnants/ aplasia)	V3 Transverse vaginal septum and/or imperforate hymen V4 Vaginal aplasia
U6 Unclassified malformations		
U		*C* *V*

Fig. 2: ESHRE/ESGE classification of female genital tract congenital anomalies.

The European Society of Human Reproduction and Embryology (ESHRE) and the European Society for Gynaecological Endoscopy (ESGE) have established in 2013 a new updated classification system using the anatomy as the main characteristic and where the cervical and vaginal anomalies are classified in independent supplementary subclasses.[7]

In this system the septate uterus is classified as class U2 and incorporates all cases with normal fusion and abnormal resorption of the midline septum. Septate is defined as the uterus with normal outline and an internal indentation at the fundal midline exceeding 50% of the uterine wall thickness. This indentation could divide partly or completely the uterine cavity including in some cases cervix and/or vagina. Class U2 is further divided into Class U2a or partial septate uterus and class U2b or complete septate uterus.

The external uterine contour may be convex, may be flat or slightly concave with a fundal minimal indentation.[8] The ASRM system does not specify the depth of the indentation for differentiate a septate from a bicornuate but a limit of 1 cm have been established. The ESHRE/ESGE classification set an external indentation under 50% of the uterine wall thickness.

It is important to note that the septate uterus can also have an associated double cervix and a double cervix with vaginal septum. Since the first case report in 1994 by McBean,[9] more than 100 cases have been published. Cervical duplication has been traditionally associated with other mullerian anomalies as didelphic uterus and probably the true incidence of septate uterus with cervical duplication is much greater than we thought.

DIAGNOSIS

Hysterosalpingography

Hysterosalpingography alone is not adequate to make the distinction between a septate and a bicornuate uterus unless the angle of divergence of two straight uterine cavities is 75 degree or less, indicating a septate uterus.[10]

Ultrasound

Transvaginal ultrasonography, hysterosonography and three-dimensional ultrasonography (3D US) can be used in the detection of a septate uterus. The sensitivity of those sonographic imaging modalities ranges between 95.21% and 99.29%.[11]

Two-dimensional ultrasound (2D US) is an acceptable method for the diagnosis of the uterine anomalies. The main limitation is the impossibility to obtain a coronal view of the uterus. The accuracy rate of 2D US in the diagnosis of uterine malformation is 80.65%. As noted above, color Doppler reveals septal vascularity in 71% of the patients.[12]

Magnetic Resonance Imaging

Magnetic resonance imaging (MRI) offers information about the uterine cavity and about the external contour of the uterus and with a reported accuracy of

100% in the diagnosis of uterine malformations when it is compared with the association laparoscopy/hysteroscopy. There is also an excellent agreement between MRI and clinical diagnosis of mullerian anomalies. The main causes of disagreement are MRI diagnosis of septate uteri with two cervices clinically diagnosed as didelphic, partial septate uteri clinically diagnosed as arcuate and complex anomalies with features of more than one class.[13]

The combination of hysteroscopy and laparoscopy is actually considered the "gold standard" for the diagnosis of the uterine malformation, as the cavity and the external aspect of the uterus can be evaluated.

TREATMENT

Hysteroscopy metroplasty is, in fact, a transverse incision of the uterine septum instead a resection. This incision has to be made in the middle of the septum, equidistant to the anterior and posterior uterine walls. Tubal ostia are helpful to maintain the right plane avoiding the inadvertent trauma to the normal myometrium.

The determination of the correct incision line is one of the most important parts of the hysteroscopic metroplasty, but this imaginary line is not always easy to determine. Levent, Yasar, Ali Suha, and Sonmez described the "Suha-Levent sign". After methylene blue injection, they found a well-defined blue line of 2–3 mm, over the septum between the tubal ostia and equidistant to the anterior and the posterior walls. This blue guide helped them to identify the correct incision line.[14]

Two different surgical approaches for the septum have been described; the thinning technique and the shortening one.[15]

In the "thinning technique", longitudinal incisions are performed over each side of the septum from the lower tip to the base at fundus. The objective is to reduce the width of the septum and to transform the initial septum in to a fundal remnant of tissue that can be incised from one cornual recess to the other. In the "shortening" technique, the septum is incised transversely, starting from the apex towards the fundus. This incision in the middle of the septum, retracts the remaining tissue towards the anterior and posterior uterine walls.

The selection of one of the above technique depends on the width and the length of the septum. For a broad septum it is better to use the thinner technique while for a thin septum, the "shortening" is the most appropriate.

The classical criteria used to decide when the metroplasty is completed and is necessary to stop the surgery are when both ostia are seen in a panoramic view and when the tip of the endoscope can move freely from one ostium towards the other.

It is well accepted after the study of Fedele that a residual septum less than 1 cm shown by ultrasonography after the hysteroscopic metroplasty does not affect to the reproductive outcomes compared with women with a complete resection.[16]

The transcervical hysteroscopic metroplasty is usually performed with monopolar or bipolar resectosope (electrosurgery), using a semicircular loop at 0 degree or a Collins knife. The use of this instrument needs a prior dilatation of the cervix. In those cases of complete septum or in case with double cervix, it is important to access both hemicavities by an appropriate dilatation of both cervical canals. In this way we can have an easier movement of the resectoscope inside uterine cavity. The use of the resectoscope is preferred in cases of complete septum, and in case of broad-vascularized septum, as electric energy provides simultaneous hemostasis.

Of late there is a preference to use the scissors for cutting the septum. This is due to a realization that use of electrosurgery on endometrium leads to more postsurgical adhesions compared to mechanical cutting. In case of a perforation, the use of electrosurgery may end up in more severe sequelae. Others prefer the use of bipolar electrode, coagulating the vessels that found during section and minimizing the bleeding during the surgery. A recent study comparing scissors and bipolar metroplasty in ambulatory setting found that the second one induces significantly higher pain scores than cold instruments. The published results of metroplasy with bipolar electrode are similar to those performed with resectoscope. The hysteroscopic treatment of septate uterus with laser is effective and safe, with minimum intraoperative bleeding.[17]

Some guidance to control the depth of the cutting of septum is helpful during the hysteroscopic metroplasty, to avoid a uterine perforation and also to achieve a complete septum resection. While some studies recommend the use of laparoscopic guidance, others believe that the ultrasound guidance have to be the method of choice even better than laparoscopy in terms of efficacy and safety.[18,19]

We believe that the use of laparoscopy may be decided in a case to case approach. A prior laparoscopy assessment generally obviates the need for current concomitant use of a laparoscopy. We have observed a much higher rate (50%) of endometriosis in cases of uterine fusion anomalies, probably due to incoordinate uterine contractions leading to higher reflux of menses. And hence in women where infertility, recurrent pregnancy Loss (RPL), and menstrual pain is a complaint, we recommend a simultaneous laparoscopy.

POSTOPERATIVE TREATMENT

The postoperative administration of estrogen hormonal therapy has been used to stimulate the endometrial growth, and to reduce the formation of intrauterine adhesions. In initial days of hysteroscopic septum resection, it was a common practice to insert an intrauterine device (IUD) after the resection. But the experience over the years and the published data have shown that the IUD is not necessary for an optimal result.[20,21] An attempt to use intrauterine bio-chemical substances to reduce the adhesion formation is also made. But, the evidence of the effectiveness of using any anti-adhesion gel in women of reproductive age treated by operative hysteroscopy for uterine septum is inconclusive till date.

REFERENCES

1. Lee DM, Osathanondh R, Yeh J. Localization of Bcl-2 in the human fetal mullerian tract. Fertil Steril. 1998;70(1):135-40.
2. Connell M, Owen C, Segars J. Genetic syndromes and genes involved in the development of the female reproductive tract : A possible role for gene therapy. J Genet Syndr Gene Ther. 2013;4. pii: 127.
3. Liatsikos SA, Grimbizis GF, Georgiou I, et al. HOX A10 and HOX A11 mutation scan in congenital malformations of the female genital tract. Reprod Biomed online. 2010;21(1):126-32.
4. Chan YY, Jayaprakasan K, Zamora J, et al. The prevalence of congenital uterine anomalies in unselected and high-risk populations: a systematic review. Hum Reprod Update. 2011;17(6):761-71.
5. Buttram VC Jr. Gibbons WE, Mullerian anomalies: a proposed classification. (An analysis of 144 cases). Fertil Steril. 1979;32(1):40-6.
6. The American Fertility Society classifications of adnexal adhesions, distal tubal occlusion, tubal occlusion secondary to tubal ligation, tubal pregnancies, mullerian anomalies and intrauterine adhesions. Fertil Steril. 1988;49(6):944-55.
7. Grimbizis GF, Gordts S, Di Spiezio Sardo A, et al. The ESHRE/ESGE consensus on the classification of female genital tract congenital anomalies. Hum Report. 2013;28(8);2032-44.
8. Troiano RN, McCarthy SM. Mullerian duct anomalies: imaging and clinical issues. Radiology. 2004;233(1):19-34.
9. McBean JH, Brumsted JR. Septate uterus with cervical duplication: a rare malformation. Fertil Steril. 1994;62(2):415-7.
10. Reuter KL, Daly DC, Cohen SM. Septate versus bicornuate uteri; errors in imaging diagnosis. Radiol. 1989;172;749-52.
11. Kupesic S, Kurjak A. Septate uterus; detection and prediction of obstetrical complications by different forms of ultrasonography. J Ultrasound Med. 1998;17(10);631-2.
12. Yu LL, Zhang X, Zhang T, et al. Detection of congenital uterine malformation by using transvaginal three-dimensional ultrasound. Journal of Huazhong University of Science and Technology Medical Sciences. 2014;34(5);782-4.
13. Mueller GC, Hussain HK, Smith YR, et al. Mullerian duct anomalies: comparison of MRI diagnosis and clinical diagnosis. AJR Am J Roentgenol. 2007;189(6);1294-8.
14. Yasar L, Sonmez AS, Savan K, et al. A practical guide to determine the incision line in the treatment of septate uterus: "Suha-Levent's Sign", Arch Gynecol Obstet. 2009;279(6);809-11.
15. Homer HA, Li TC, Cooke ID. The septate uterus; a review of management and reproductive outcome. Fertil Sterility. 2000;73(1);1-14.
16. Fedele L, Bianchi S, Marchini M, et al. Residual uterine septum of less than 1cm after hysteroscopic metroplasty does not impair reproductive outcome. Hum Reprod. 1996;11(4); 727-9.
17. Kamel MAM, El-Tawab SS, El-Ashkar OS, et al. Mini-Scissor Versus Bipolar Twizzle in Ambulatory Hysteroscopic Metroplasty: A Prospective Randomized Study. J Gynecol Surg. 2014;30(3); 147-51.
18. Litta P, Pozzan C, Merlin F, et al. Hysteroscopic metroplasty under laparoscopic guidance in infertile women with septate uteri: follow-up of reproductive outcome. J Reprod Med. 2004;49(4):274-8.
19. Coccia ME, Becattini C, Bracco GL, et al. Intraoperative ultrasound guidance for operative hysteroscopy. A prospective study. J Reprod Med. 2000;45(5):413-8.
20. Dabirashrafi H, Mohammed K, Moghadami-Tabrizi N, et al. Is estrogen necessary after hysteroscopic incision of the uterine septum? The Journal of the American Association of Gynecologic Laparoscopists. 1996;3(4):623-5.
21. Nawroth F, Schmidt T, Freise C, et al. Is it possible to recommend an "optimal" postoperative management after hysteroscopic metroplasty? A retrospective study with 52 infertile patients showing a septate uterus. Acta Obstet Gynecol Scand. 2002;81(1):55-7.

Chapter 11

Complications of Hysteroscopic Surgery

Sujata Kar

INTRODUCTION

Hysteroscopy is a minimally invasive gynecological procedure. The development of new hysteroscopic instruments, fiber optics, and digital video equipment has continued to provide more varied, efficacious, and less invasive procedures. The introduction of smaller-diameter hysteroscopes has allowed operative hysteroscopy to become a predominantly office and outpatient procedure. As with any procedure, this also has a few complications. 2.7–3.8% of all hysteroscopies,[1] 0.13% in diagnostic hysteroscopy, 0.96% in operative hysteroscopy,[2] highest rate of complications seen with hysteroscopic adhesiolysis—4.5% (Fig. 1). These complications are broadly classified into the following points.

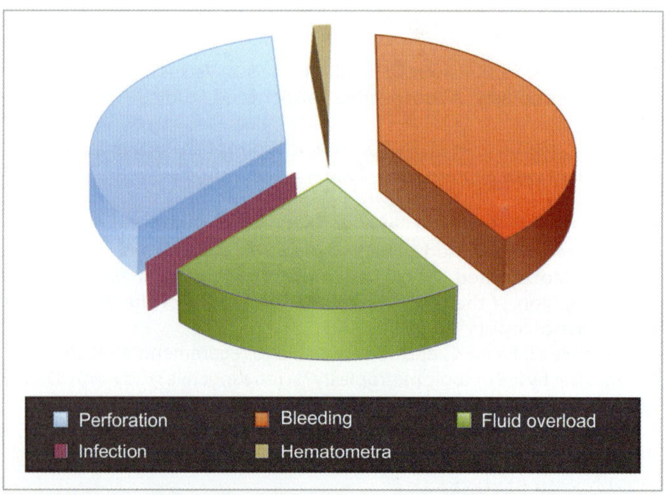

Fig. 1: Hysteroscopic complications.

MECHANICAL OR TRAUMATIC COMPLICATIONS

These types of complications are among the most common. Other categories include preoperative complications (i.e. improper patient selection and lack of informed consent), electrosurgical and gaseous, complications related to distention media, and postoperative complications (i.e. infection and late sequelae).

Inability to Insert the Hysteroscope

Causes: Stenotic, nulliparous cervix, menopause, GnRH agonists, previous cone biopsy, laceration, or cryosurgery; or an acutely retroflexed or anteflexed uterus.

Prevention

- Acute flexion problems can be corrected using a long-bladed, open-sided Graves speculum deep in the anterior or posterior fornix. The speculum pushes the fundus to the mid-position and facilitates dilation. Once the hysteroscope is inserted, remove the speculum.
- Placing a tenaculum on the posterior lip of the cervix of an acutely retroflexed uterus will straighten the cervical canal when traction is applied.
- Inserting a laminaria tent the evening before surgery helps dilate the cervix easily and atraumatically. However, the laminaria can sometimes create a false passage, leading to perforation.
- Cervical ripening agents such as intravaginal or oral misoprostol (200 µg inserted vaginally or 400 µg orally 8–12 hours preoperatively) also can facilitate dilation.
- Intracervical injection of vasopressin solution (4 IU in 100 cc sodium chloride, injected at the 4 o'clock and 8 o'clock positions) can reduce the force needed to dilate the cervix. Half-size dilators may help; they also reduce the risk of cervical laceration.

Laceration of the Cervix

Although this is a minor complication, substantial bleeding sometimes occurs, when the cervix is lacerated by the tenaculum. Bleeding from lower uterus or cervical canal can obscure view. In some cases, bleeding is delayed, necessitating additional surgery. Intravasation of distention fluid also can occur at these lacerations.

In these cases,

1. Suture the cervix
2. Occasionally, a touch of cautery from the roller ball electrode at low power (20–30 W) can control the bleeding.
3. Silver nitrate sticks or ferric subsulfate (Monsel's) paste are also effective on superficial lacerations.
   Coagulation with the electrode may be necessary when bleeding is heavy.

Creating a False Passage (Fig. 2)

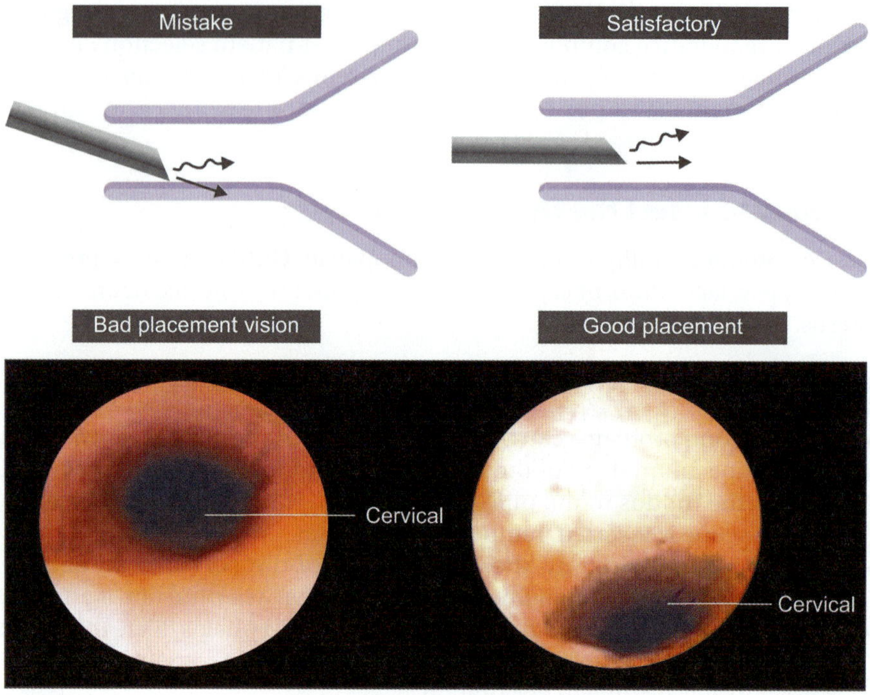

Fig. 2: Representation of cervical canal.

Uterine Perforation (Fig. 3)

Uterine perforation may occur during cervical dilatation, hysteroscope insertion, and intramyometrial tissue resection. In particular, the risk of perforation increases in case of fibroids with intramural component when an aggressive uterine fibroid resection into the myometrium is carried out.[3,4]

In case of uterine perforation, the procedure should be terminated immediately and, if there is a mechanical perforation in which bowel damage is not suspected, the patient can be observed and discharged if stable.[5]

If a perforation occurs secondarily to an activated electrode then it should be assumed that there is a bowel injury until proven otherwise, and laparoscopy must be done without delay.[5]

ELECTROSURGICAL AND GASEOUS COMPLICATIONS

Most electrosurgical complications involve activation of an electrode at the time of perforation, or current diversion to the outer sheath. Thermal injuries also can be caused by overheating of the return pad or use of a hot speculum after removal from the autoclave. The latter can be avoided by immersing the entire speculum in cool saline for at least 1–2 minutes prior to inserting it into

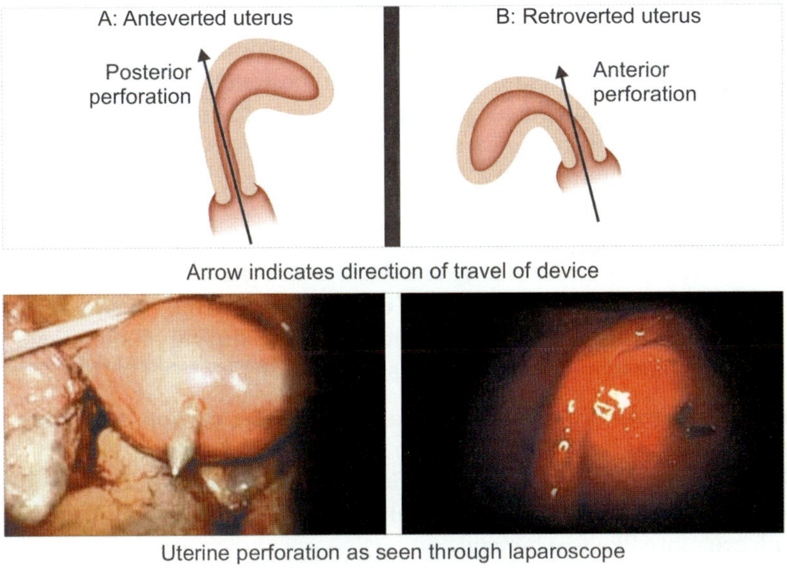

Fig. 3: Uterine perforation.

the vagina. The blade cools much faster than the weighted ball, so be sure to check both to prevent a perineal or buttock burn.

Perforation with an active electrode usually occurs when current is applied as the electrode is extended or the resectoscope is moved toward the fundus. It can be avoided if the electrode is activated only when moving it toward the operator.

Perforations with intraabdominal burns also have occurred during attempts to coagulate bleeders—especially in the cornual regions.

Diversion of current can be destructive. Genital tract injuries have occurred as a result of current diversion. The usual cause: electrode insulation failure, which allows current to jump to the outer sheath of the resectoscope. To avoid this, inspect all electrodes thoroughly before surgery and use them only once.

Capacitative coupling also diverts current. Since the sheath-within-a-sheath design of the resectoscope resembles a capacitor, high-voltage current can jump to the outer sheath without direct contact from the electrode. One way to avoid these injuries is to activate the electrode intermittently, with short bursts, rather than rolling back and forth over an area with continuous current.

Another strategy is placing a damp sponge in the posterior vagina extending out the introitus; this protects the mucosa and perineal skin—especially in obese patients.

How to Avoid Return-pad Injuries

Keep the patient's thigh completely dry; ensure that the pad is flat against the skin at application, with no bubbles or creases; and use only return electrode monitor (REM) dispersive pads. Especially when using vaporization electrodes, avoid prolonged activation of the electrode at high power. To minimize risk of vaporization, use a second dispersive pad connected to the first via a "y" connector to further disperse current and heat at the return pad. Also, limit the use of coagulation current and use a maximum generator setting of 60–80 W in the coagulation mode.

GAS EMBOLISM

Initial reports of this potentially fatal complication came mostly from laser ablation procedures, but gas embolism can occur during all diagnostic and operative hysteroscopic procedures, especially the latter.

Sources of gas embolism: Room air, carbon dioxide, carbon monoxide, and other gaseous products of vaporization or tissue combustion.

The anesthesiologist is usually the first to identify the signs. Carbon dioxide is a soluble gas, so these emboli generally resolve rapidly. In contrast, room air emboli are more likely to be fatal.

Signs of gas embolism: Sudden fall in oxygen saturation, as well as to hypotension, hypercarbia, arrhythmias, tachypnea, or a "mill wheel" murmur.

Treatment: If gas embolism is suspected, stop the procedure and ventilate the patient with 100% oxygen.

Prevention:

- Avoid the Trendelenburg position.
- Leave the last dilator in the cervix until just before inserting the resectoscope.
- Limit repetitive removal and reinsertion of the resectoscope, as often occurs during myoma resection.
- By vaporizing rather than resecting myomas, it is possible to eliminate the need to continually remove fibroid chips.
- Preoperative GnRH agonists narrow venous sinuses and help prevent this complication.
- Intracervical injection of dilute vasopressin prior to dilatation of the cervix creates vascular spasm and may help prevent gas from entering the circulation.

COMPLICATIONS FROM DISTENTION MEDIA

Excess absorption of distention media is one of the most frequent complications. Most surgeons use low-viscosity, sodium-free fluids for operative hysteroscopy, since fluids that contain electrolytes are incompatible with monopolar electrosurgical instruments. The use of 3% sorbitol, 1.5% glycine, or sorbitol-mannitol solutions can lead to dilutional hyponatremia and hypoosmolality. Although the vast majority of women quickly recover from these conditions, some cases of permanent morbidity and even death have been reported. The overall incidence of dilutional hyponatremia was 0.2% in 1993.

Severe fluid overload can cause pulmonary edema, hyponatremia, heart failure, cerebral edema and even death. Fluid absorption occurs through the open veins of the fibroid and possibly through transperitoneal absorption from retrograde flow through the Fallopian tubes.

Guidelines indicate that fluid intravasation of 750 mL during surgery requires planned termination of the operation and that the intervention must be immediately stopped when balance exceeds of 1,000 mL or, 1,500–2,000 mL.

The risk factors for intravasation during hysteroscopic myomectomy are not completely elucidated because no studies have tested their independent contribution or relation to fluid loss.

Factors associated with a higher risk of intravasation

Most important—Intramural extension of the fibroid; indeed, in cases of fibroids with deep intramural extension, intravasation will increase mainly because of damage to larger-sized vessels, also length of the operation, the size of the fibroid and the total inflow volume.

Management of this risk relies on close monitoring of the fluid balance and interruption of the procedure before excessive fluid absorption occurs. The difference between the amount of inflow and outflow fluid (including also fluid leaking from the vagina) could be assessed by dedicated operating room personnel or by modern electronic balances and pumps (i.e. Hydromat Gyn and Equimat, Karl Storz GmbH Co., Tuttlingen, Germany; HysteroBalance/ HysteroFlow, Olympus Medical System GmbH, Hamburg, Germany).

Prevention: The use of normal saline combined with bipolar energy reduces the risk of hyponatremia (eliminating the problem of the accumulation of the free water), but an excessive intravasation (1,500 mL) still remains a risk and might cause cardiac overload.

LONG-TERM COMPLICATIONS OF HYSTEROSCPIC SURGERY

Postoperative intrauterine adhesions represents the major long-term complication of hysterosocpic myomectomy and other major hysteroscopic surgeries; ranging from 1% to 13%.

Prevention

- Avoid forced cervical manipulation, and trauma of healthy endometrium and myometrium surrounding the fibroid.
- Reduce the usage of electrosurgery especially during the removal of fibroids with extensive intramural involvement and multiple fibroids on opposing endometrial surfaces

- An early second-look hysteroscopy after any hysteroscopic surgery is another effective preventive and therapeutic strategy.
- Pharmacologic (conjugated estrogen, levonorgestrel releasing intrauterine device) and barrier agents, including Foley catheter, hyaluronic acid gel and hyaluronic acid and carboxymethyl cellulose (Seprafilm).
- A recent review has clearly indicated that there is no single modality proven to be unequivocally effective at preventing postoperative adhesion formation for hysteroscopic surgery.

Uterine perforation in a subsequent pregnancy: It is a rare but possible late complication. Possible risk factors are perforation during surgery, large myoma, short duration between surgery and subsequent pregnancy.

Iatrogenic adenomyosis: Two theories suggest this is a late complication of operative hysteroscopy. According to the first, when the endometrium is incompletely resected, scarring over this tissue causes the viable glands to grow into the myometrium. The other theory suggests that viable endometrial debris is transported into the myometrium by vessels opened at resection.

Hematometra: This can occur following operative hysteroscopy if viable glands are left in the fundal or cornual region and synechiae develop in the lower segment, preventing egress of blood. It also can occur if the upper endocervix is ablated and subsequently scars, causing stenosis.

To avoid this, ablate only to the level of the internal os. Hematometra can be diagnosed easily by ultrasound and treated with office hysteroscopy using a narrow-diameter, rigid, continuous-flow hysteroscope with an operating channel to pass small instruments.

CONCLUSION

To avoid complications it is important to know the *contraindications* for hysteroscopic surgery:

- Unfamiliarity with equipment, instruments, or technique
- Lack of appropriate equipment or staff familiar with the equipment
- Acute pelvic inflammatory disease
- Pregnancy
- Genital tract malignancies
- Lack of informed consent
- Inability to dilate the cervix
- Inability to distend the uterus to obtain visualization
- Poor surgical candidates who may not tolerate fluid overload because of renal disease, or radiofrequency current when a cardiac pacemaker is present.

REFERENCES

1. Propst AM, Liberman RF, Harlow BL, et al. Complications of hysteroscopic surgery: predicting patients at risk. Obstet Gynecol. 2000;96:517-20.
2. Jansen FW, Van Dongen H, Emanuel MH, et al. Follow-up after incomplete hysteroscopic removal of uterine fibroids. Acta Obstet Gynecol Scand. 2006;85:1463-7.
3. Mazzon I, Cittadini E, Perino A, et al. Nuova tecnica per la miometomia isteroscopica: enucleazione con ansa fredda, Testo-Atlante di Chirurgia Endoscopica Ginecologica. 1995. Palermo, Italy COFESE Ed cap XXXIIIb.
4. Murakami T, Tamura M, Ozawa Y, et al. Safe techniques in surgery for hysteroscopic myomectomy. J Obstet Gynaecol Res. 2005;31:216-23.
5. Indman PD. Hysteroscopic treatment of submucous fibroids. Clin Obstet Gynecol. 2006;49:811-20.

Chapter 12

Hysteroscopic Contraception

Polly Chatterjee

INTRODUCTION

A WHO survey in 1992 estimated that about 100 million women rely on permanent sterilization as a form of contraception. A 1995 survey of several thousand US women found that the most popular contraceptive methods for a couple were female surgical sterilization (28%) and oral contraceptives (27%). The Royal College of Obstetricians and Gynaecologists survey in 1999 estimated that in approximately 30% of couples with at least one partner sterilized, female sterilization was more popular than male sterilization.

Transcervical sterilization was initially attempted in the 19th century and a variety of techniques have been assessed in an attempt to provide an alternative to traditional sterilization methods. In 1934, Schroeder first performed direct visualization of the tubal ostia using electrosurgery. Three modalities have been used: chemical agents, electrodiathermy and mechanical methods. Electrosurgical sterilization was found to have a high morbidity and has been abandoned. Of the chemical agents, quinacrine has shown the most promising results and is still under investigation. A variety of mechanical or occlusive plugs were poorly retained.

Essure, a new female sterilization method approved by the US Food and Drug Administration (FDA), offers women a new option for controlling fertility. The technique is done without an incision, is hormone-free, and can be performed on an outpatient basis under local anesthesia. There are few or no side effects.

The device is a metal and polymer micro-insert 4 cm long and 1 to 2 mm wide when deployed (Fig. 1). It consists of an inner coil of stainless and polyethylene terephthalate (steel PET) fibers and a super elastic coil of nickel-titanium (nitinol). It comes loaded in a single-use delivery system. The effectiveness is believed to be due to the space filling design of the device coupled with a local occlusive, benign tissue response to the PET fibers that result in device retention and pregnancy prevention.

A polymer matrix implant, Adiana, was approved in 2009, but was withdrawn by the manufacturer in 2012 because of high failure rates.

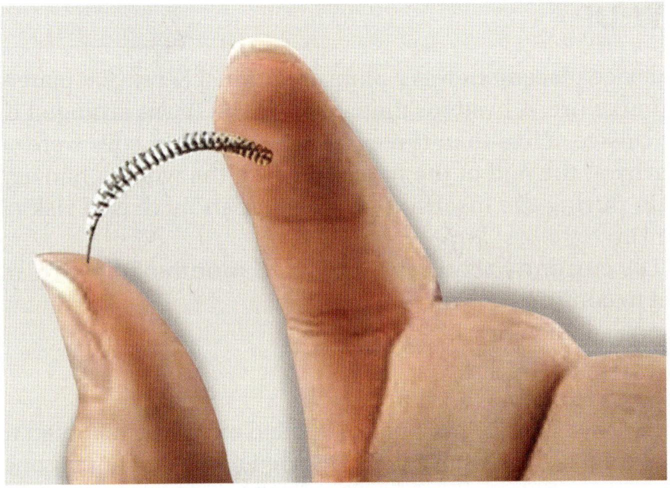

Fig. 1: Essure: a new female sterilization device.

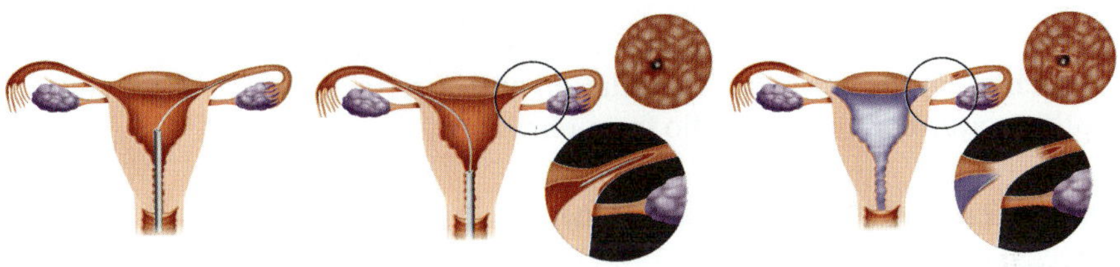

Fig. 2: Step-by-step method of Essure application.

METHOD

The procedure is done in the first half of the menstrual cycle. A premedication of diclofenac sodium 100 mg and paracetamol 1 g orally 2 hours prior to their appointment was enough. If non-steroidal inflammatory agents were contraindicated, 30 mg of codeine phosphate was substituted.

The vaginosocopic approach of hysteroscopy without the use of local anesthetic is the normal procedure. Three liter bags of normal saline in a pressure bag set at 60–100 mm Hg were used for irrigation. A standard hysteroscope with a 5 Fr operating channel is enough. *Rescue* analgesia, by way of *Entonox*, was available if required. Women could watch the procedure on the monitor if they wished and were allowed home within 30 min of the procedure. Two nurses were required in the clinic: one to attend to the patient and the other to assist the surgeon and monitor the irrigation fluid (Fig. 2).

FOLLOW-UP

Check of device placement was a plain abdominal X-ray (flat plate) 3 months after the procedure. A hysterosalpingogram (HSG) was arranged if the X-ray was inconclusive, if less than three or more than eight coils were seen in the uterine cavity at the end of the procedure or if the women had experienced undue pain during the insertion (suggesting an increased risk of possible perforation).

The FDA currently requires a HSG at 3 months following the Essure placement to confirm tubal occlusion.

POTENTIAL RISKS

- The micro-inserts may have been expelled out of the fallopian tubes.
- The coil implants may have been inserted too far, or not far enough, into the fallopian tubes.
- The micro-inserts may have been pushed through the uterus or fallopian tube wall (perforation). Should this occur, surgery may be needed to repair the situation.
- The coil implants could become damaged during other medical procedures, such as endometrial biopsy, dilation and curettage (D&C), or procedures that require the use of radio frequency.

Complications during Insertion

- Mild-to-moderate pain
- Nausea and vomiting
- Fainting following the procedure
- Undiagnosed pregnancy
- Infection.

ESSURE EFFECTIVENESS

Research has shown that less than 1.7 out of every 1,000 women end up becoming pregnant 5 years after the procedure (99.83% effective).

By the 3-month follow-up perform HSG test:

- Approximately, 1% of women may have one of the coil implants missing.
- 96% of women's fallopian tubes will have been successfully blocked.

By 6 months after the procedure, 100% of women should have both tubes fully closed.

COMPARISON WITH LAPAROSCOPIC STERILIZATION: EFFECTIVENESS AND RISKS

Laparoscopic sterilization is an invasive abdominal procedure associated with recognized complications. A prospective study of the complications of diagnostic laparoscopy by Kane and Krejs revealed rates of 5.1% for minor complications and 2.3% for major complications requiring surgery or transfusion. The US Collaborative Review of Sterilization (CREST) study showed that the risk of laparotomy to complete the sterilization procedure is greater if the woman has a history of previous abdominal or pelvic surgery or obesity greater than 12% of ideal body weight.

Essure offers an alternative choice for patients with some medical conditions like cardiopulmonary disease, autoimmune disorders and genetic disorders, congenital heart disease contraindicate laparoscopic sterilization under general anesthesia.

A lower failure rate has been obtained with the Filshie clip. A prospective 10-year follow-up study using the Filshie clip was commenced at the Family Planning Association in Nottingham in 1982 and only one patient out of 434 became pregnant giving a lifetime risk of 2.5 per 1,000.

The CREST study reported a 10-year failure rate of 2% in the laparoscopic approach of sterilization. A 10-year retrospective review of pregnancy data in Essure cases revealed 748 pregnancies in 4,97,305 patients or a 99.4% effectiveness rate.

COUNSELING

Women opting for the Essure should be advised of the absolute irreversibility of the procedure, a 5–10% insertion failure rate, possible complications of uterine perforation, device migration and infection. It was emphasized that they would be required to continue to use contraception until a check abdominal X-ray or HSG was done at 3 months post procedure. High vaginal and cervical swabs were taken routinely and cervical cytology when indicated.

Finally, clinicians may be more wary of the complete irreversibility of the procedure. It is of course vital that patients are fully counseled prior to any sterilization operation, but some women may still regret the decision at a later date. The full range of contraceptive options should be discussed along with the attendant medical and surgical risks, risk of failure and alternatives.

Successful in vitro fertilization pregnancies have now been reported after Essure (AAGL Nov. 2004) when micro-inserts were used to obstruct tubes distally obstructed by a hydrosalpinx prior to assisted fertility treatment.

Women having menorrhagia can be treated with endometrial ablation, transcervical resection of myoma (TCRM) or polyp at the same sitting.

COST

A possible reason for the slow uptake of Essure is the cost of the devices; a pair of Essure devices costs around £550, whereas two Filshie clips cost £140. When staff, theatre time, in-patient costs, administration and other hospital charges are taken into account, the costs per treatment are rather closer with laparoscopic sterilization with Filshie clips costing £714.64 per treatment and Essure hysteroscopic sterilization £816.46. An American cost-analysis study found office hysteroscopic placement of the Essure device to be a more cost-effective method than laparoscopic tubal ligation.

CONCLUSION

Essure hysteroscopic sterilization is a simple, reproducible procedure that, after appropriate training, can be performed by any gynecologist with experience in outpatient hysteroscopy. Women requesting permanent contraception should now have the choice of this outpatient procedure. It avoids the risks of laparoscopic sterilization and the 5-year results are promising.

In a recent cohort controlled comparative study of Essure versus laparoscopic sterilization Duffy et al. showed that Essure hysteroscopic sterilization is associated with greater patient satisfaction than laparoscopic sterilization.

Over 50,000 procedures have been performed worldwide to date, with 12,000 of these in Europe. NICE guidance on the Essure procedure in 2004 concluded that units performing Essure hysteroscopic sterilization must have special arrangements for audit or research due to lack of availability of long term details.

FURTHER READING

1. Bayer Pharmaceuticals. Available at: http://www.essure.com/. Accessed December 2017.
2. Brito LG, Cohen SL, Goggins ER, et al. Essure surgical removal and subsequent symptom resolution: case series and follow-up survey. J Minim Invasive Gynecol. 2015;22:910-3.
3. Chern B, Siow A. Initial Asian experience in hysteroscopic sterilisation using the Essure permanent birth control device. BJOG. 2005;112(9):1322-7
4. Chudnoff SG, Nichols JE Jr, Levie M. Hysteroscopic Essure inserts for permanent contraception: extended follow-up results of a phase III multicenter international study. J Minim Invasive Gynecol. 2015;22:951.
5. Cleary TP, Tepper NK, Cwiak C, et al. Pregnancies after hysteroscopic sterilization: a systematic review. Contraception. 2013;87:539.
6. Cooper JM, Carignan CS, Cher D, et al. Selective tubal occlusion procedure 2000 investigators group. Microinsert nonincisional hysteroscopic sterilisation. Obstet Gynaecol. 2003;102(1):59-67.
7. Department of Health website. (2005). UK (2004–2005) Hospital episode statistics. [online] Available from http://www. hesonline.nhs.uk. [Accessed December 2017].
8. Dhruva SS, Ross JS, Gariepy AM. Revisiting Essure-toward safe and effective sterilization. N Engl J Med. 2015;373:e17.
9. Hitzerd E, Schreuder HW, Vleugels MP, et al. Twelve year retrospective review of unintended pregnancies after Essure sterilization in the Netherlands. Fertil Steril. 2016;105:932-7.
10. Jamieson DJ, Hillis SD, Duerr A, et al. Complications of interval laparoscopic tubal sterilization: findings from the United States Collaborative Review of Sterilization. Obstet Gynecol. 2000;96:997.
11. Jones J, Mosher W, Daniels K. (2012) National Health Statistics Report: Current Contraceptive Use in the United States, 2006–2010, and Changes in Patterns of Use Since 1995. [online] Available from http://www.cdc. gov/nchs/data/nhsr/nhsr060.pdf. Accessed December 2017.
12. Kane MG, Krejs GJ. Complications of diagnostic laparoscopy in Dallas: a 7-year prospective study. Gastrointest Endosc. 1984;30:237-40
13. Kerin JF, Munday DN, Ritossa MG, et al. Essure hysteroscopic sterilisation: results based on new coil catheter delivery system. J Am J Gynaecol Laparosc. 2004;11(3):388-93.
14. Peterson HB, Xia Z, Hughes JM, et al. The risk of pregnancy after tubal sterilisation: Findings from the US collaborative review of sterilisation. Am J Obstet Gynaecol. 1996;174:1161-70.

15. Peterson HB, Xia Z, Hughes JM, et al. The risk of pregnancy after tubal sterilization: findings from the U.S. Collaborative Review of Sterilization. Am J Obstet Gynecol. 1996;174:1161.
16. Royal College of Obstetricians and Gynaecologists. (1999) National evidence based guidelines: Male and female sterilisation. London: RCOG.
17. Trussell J, Guilbert E, Hedley A. Sterilization failure, sterilization reversal, and pregnancy after sterilization reversal in Quebec. Obstet Gynecol. 2003;101:677.
18. Ubeda A, Labastida R, Dexeus S. Essure: a new device for hysteroscopic tubal sterilization in an outpatient setting. Fertil Steril. 2004;82(1):196-9.
19. US Food and Drug administration. (2005). PMA final decisions rendered for July 2005. Available from http://www.fda.gov/cdrh/pma/ pmajul05.html. [Accessed December 2017].
20. US Food and Drug Administration. (2015) Update on the status of FDA's evaluation of the Essure System.[online] Available from http://www.fda.gov/MedicalDevices/ProductsandMedical Procedures/ImplantsandProsthetics/ EssurePermanentBirthControl/ucm473946.htm. [Accessed December 2017].
21. World Health Organisation. Female sterilisation. A guide to provision of services. New York Health Organisation. 1992.